Sex and Gender Differences in Health and Disease

Sex and Gender Differences in Health and Disease

Ricky L. Langley, MD, MPH

CAROLINA ACADEMIC PRESS
Durham, North Carolina

Copyright © 2003
Ricky L. Langley
All Rights Reserved

ISBN 0-89089-471-X
LCCN 2003106137

CAROLINA ACADEMIC PRESS
700 Kent Street
Durham, North Carolina 27701
Telephone (919) 489-7486
Fax (919)493-5668
www.cap-press.com

Printed in the United States of America

Contents

Preface	vii
Introduction	ix
Dermatology	3
Neurology	37
Cardiology	63
Pulmonology	101
Endocrinology/Metabolism	115
Nephrology/Urology	135
Allergy/Immunology	151
Hematology/Oncology	157
Gastroenterology	173
Orthopedics/Rheumatology	195
Reproductive Health	227
Infectious Diseases	237
Ophthalmology	251
Otolaryngology	261
Dental Health	271
Psychiatry	277
Behavioral and Psychological Health	295
Pharmacology/Toxicology	305
Other/Miscellaneous	321
References	329

Preface

Are there differences in health and diseases between males and females? Obviously there are some physical differences, primarily in the reproductive organs, that distinguish males from females. But are the other organs anatomically and functionally the same in males and females? Do diseases manifest the same? Are medications equally efficacious? Do side effects from medications differ? Do hormones play any role in how diseases manifest in men versus women? Are some diseases (besides those of the reproductive organs) more common in one sex and if so why?

These are just a few questions that this book will attempt to address. This book is arranged by body system. Within each body system, normal anatomical and physiological differences between males and females are presented. Additionally, normal laboratory value differences between males and females are provided.

Differences in disease prevalence or manifestations are discussed by body system. Information is provided on which sex has an higher disease prevalence, the ratio of disease prevalence in males to females when it could be found, and occasionally interesting facts about different manifestations of the disease between the sexes. In certain diseases, the prevalence may be similar, but the disease may manifest differently or be more severe in one sex and this is also noted.

This book also includes a section on pharmacological and toxicological differences on how the sexes respond to medications or environmental agents. For example, the half-life and clearance of a drug may differ when administered to a male or female. Why does this difference occur? In many cases, it is unknown why, but new research is finding differences in the amounts or types of enzymes in the body which probably accounts for some of this difference.

In the final chapter, miscellaneous topics are presented that do not fit neatly into a specific body system. However, these are differences that have been frequently noted between the sexes.

This book should be of interest to physicians, geneticists, anatomists, physiologists, pharmacologists, epidemiologists, toxicologists and others interested in differences in anatomy, physiology, and disease occurrence between the sexes. It can also be used as a resource for teachers of gender studies courses. Hopefully this book will spark interest and research in finding out why differences between the sexes occur in so many diseases.

Introduction

Gender-Based Biology

A new field of interest, gender-based biology, identifies physiological and biological differences between women and men at the subcellular, cellular, tissue, organ, and system level and the effects of pharmaceutical agents on males and females. It is known that women in the United States live on average 7 years longer than men. The average male lifespan today is 74 years, but for females it is 81 years. Why does this difference exist? The average sex ratio at birth is 106 males for every 100 females. Over the last 20–30 years this difference has been decreasing. Is environmental pollution partly responsible? Do male and female fetuses respond differently to these pollutants which may be found in their mother's body? Certain antidepressants appear to be more effective in men versus women. Are there differences in the cytochrome enzyme systems that may explain this? Findings from gender-based biology research may help explain these differences and lead to new treatments for diseases that may vary depending upon one's sex.

Sex versus Gender

While many scientists use these terms interchangeably, there is a difference in meaning. The normal development of humans depends on the compatibility between sex chromosomes (genetic sex), sex of the gonads, internal and external genitalia formation, somatic body characteristics, and psychic sex. The psychic sex is frequently called gender and consists of gender identity (identification of self as male or female), gender role (the aspects of behavior in which males and females differ from one another in our culture at this time) and sexual orientation (heterosexual or homosexual or bisexual) and cognition (sexually dimorphic cognitive abilities). In short, the physical difference is called sex, influenced by genes and biology; the psychological difference is called gender, in which environment, cultural, and psychosocial factors have a prominent role.

Sex and Gender Differences in Illness/Injury

Studies have shown that women experience more illnesses than men, despite the fact that they live on average several years longer than men. Why does this difference exist? Is it all biological or are there other possible explanations? Women also respond to illness differently and use more health services than men. A difference in the pattern of symptom reporting exists between men and women in many surveys. This difference may indicate that women have more symptoms; women recognize symptoms more readily because they are better informed about health problems; or women may be more likely to acknowledge and report their problems. Women's experiences of menstruation, pregnancy and childbirth, and menopause cause them to think more about their bodies, their bodily sensations, and their health in ways often different from men. This may partially explain the greater frequency of visits to medical practitioners.

Researchers, including biologists, sociologists, and anthropologists, have attempted to explain some of the reasons why differences in illness occur. Sociological explanations often focus on life style differences. For example, females may be treated as the weaker sex in some countries and their medical concerns may be downplayed or ignored. Limited financial resources may limit access to health care facilities. Women's role as the primary care giver of the children may have both positive and negative impacts on her health. If the woman stays at home to raise her family, she may have less exposure to occupational hazards such as chemicals in the workplace. On the other hand, she may have higher exposure to household indoor air pollutants. She may also have less contact with people with whom she may be able to vent her worries and frustrations.

Differences in behaviors may also play a role in differences in prevalence of disease. Males tend to be risk takers, smokers, and consume alcohol more heavily than women. Men tend to be more reluctant to embrace prevention strategies. This has contributed to the spread of AIDS and other sexually transmitted diseases. Dietary differences, with women consuming less protein and calcium, may contribute to anemia and increased osteoporosis risk in females.

Occupational and recreational preferences often vary between men and women. Males are frequently involved in more outdoor activities that may increase their risk of exposure to vectors that transmit infectious agents. Males also tend to be involved in recreational activities that increase their risk of traumatic injuries such as football and bull riding.

Besides these social and lifestyle issues, that may affect one's risk of illness or injury, there are also genetic factors that may determine the risk of disease. Scientists know that autistic diseases are sex-linked and are likely to appear more in one sex (usually male). This will be discussed further below.

Technological and medical advances may have an impact on the outcome of disease treatment between the sexes. For years, females were excluded from drug trials, partly due to the fear of adverse fetal outcomes if the female would happen to become pregnant while on an investigational drug. It was often assumed (occasionally incorrectly) that females would respond to the drug the same as males. However, females today are now more likely to be included in drug trials and the results of these trials may show that females react similarly or differently to a drug. Likewise, some surgical treatments may be more technically difficult on females due to smaller organ or blood vessel size. This may cause more surgical complications and lead to increased morbidity or mortality rates in females. As surgical techniques improve, one may note the complication rate differences between the sexes to lessen.

Genetic Disorders

Genetic disorders fall into one of these categories: Chromosomal disorders; Mendelian or simple inherited disorders; and multifactorial disorders. Chromosomal disorders involve abnormal arrangement, deletion, or addition of chromosomal material. Mendelian disorders are due to mutation in a gene. Mendelian disorders display patterns of inheritance that involve the autosomes or sex chromosomes (X and Y), and are classified as dominant or recessive modes of inheritance. Most common disorders such as hypertension and heart disease are multifactorial in etiology. As the name implies, multifactorial disorders are caused by interaction of multiple genes and multiple exogenous factors.

As this book is concerned with sex differences, X-linked chromosome disorders are of concern. There are at least 350 X-linked genetic disorders known, the majority of which are recessive. X-linked recessive disorders affect males, whereas female carriers are usually spared. This is due in part to random inactivation of one of the two X-chromosomes in all female somatic cells. Thus, in female carriers of an X-linked mutation, on average 50% of the cells have the normal allele on the active X-chromosome. These functionally normal cells are usually sufficient to avoid or markedly lessen the clinical effects of an X-linked disorder in females.

How does X-linked recessive inheritance work? Usually the female sex chromosomes of an unaffected carrier mother have one faulty gene and one normal gene. The father has normal genes on the X and Y chromosomes. The resulting risk of developing the disorder in the male and female offspring are as follows: For males, there is a 50% risk of the disorder and 50% chance of being normal. For females, there is a 50% risk of being a carrier like the mother and a 50% chance of being normal.

Parent	Carrier mother Xx		Normal father Xy	
Offspring	Xx Carrier female	xy Disorder male	XX Normal female	Xy Normal male

If the male is affected and marries a normal female, then all of the female children are carriers, but the male children are normal.

Parent	Normal female XX		Disorder male xy	
Offspring	Xx Carrier female	Xx Carrier female	Xy Normal male	Xy Normal male

In X-linked recessive disorders, female children are only affected if an affected male fathers a child of a female carrier.

Parent	Carrier female Xx	Disorder male xy

Offspring	Xx	xx	Xy	xy
	Carrier female	Disorder female	Normal male	Disorder male

Dominant X-linked disorders are rare. Affected mothers transmit to one half her sons and one half her daughters. Affected fathers transmit to all daughters and no sons. The disorder tends to be less severe in heterozygous affected females than the hemizygous affected males. In some X-linked dominant disorders, there is lethality in the hemizygous male fetus. Characteristics of these dominant X-linked disorders include: The disorder occurs only in females heterozygous for the mutation; affected mothers transmit to one half of her daughters; and increased frequency of abortions occur in affected women, the abortions being of affected male fetuses.

Non-Genetic Disorders

Many differences in illnesses between males and females may be explained by non-genetic mechanisms. Exposure to various risks often differs between males and females. Males are often more likely to be risk takers, and accidental injuries and deaths are usually more prevalent in males as well as homicides.

The nature of one's work and hobbies also may put one sex or the other at increased risk. For example, hunters, primarily males, are more likely to be exposed to disease carrying insects and thus are more likely to have a higher prevalence of certain insect-transmitted diseases. Females are more likely to perform secretarial work such as typing. This may increase the females' chances of developing carpal tunnel syndrome.

Economic status may also play a role especially in third world countries where females may have jobs that pay substantially less. As a result, the type of food that can be purchased may be of lower quality and the female may be more likely to suffer from nutritional deficiencies. Housing conditions may be poorer and the female may be more likely to be exposed to weather-related problems such as heat or cold stress.

Lifestyle behaviors also may be different between males and females and partially explain some of the difference seen. Males tend to smoke, drink, and use more illicit substances than females. Males are also more likely to have medical disorders related to the abuse of these products.

However, females are increasingly using these products and are rapidly catching up with men in some disease categories such as lung cancer from tobacco use.

Multifactorial Influences

Many diseases are determined by multiple genes and their subsequent interaction with environmental factors. We know that hypertension may be due to the interaction of several different genes. Salt intake may exacerbate blood pressure changes in certain individuals with hypertension. The effects of environmental agents on various genes and the resultant adverse effect, if any, are becoming better known through advances in molecular research. Scientists are aware of many chemical agents that may form DNA adducts in the human body. The concern is that certain cancers may result due to these interactions. Certain exogenous agents may act as promoters instead of initiators of carcinogenesis. Other agents may act as teratogens causing birth defects. Research has also shown that exposure to various forms of radiation may induce illness in humans. Certain individuals with genetic defects (xeroderma pigmentosum) do not tolerate ultraviolet rays from the sun and are very susceptible to developing skin cancers from sun exposure. A growing field of inquiry is the effect endocrine disruptors may have on fetal and postnatal development in humans. As we learn more about the interactions of genes, gene proteins, and environmental agents, we may begin to get a better understanding of why differences in the prevalence of certain diseases occur between the sexes.

Sex and Gender Differences in Health and Disease

Dermatology

Anatomy and Physiology

Males have a more square shaped face, a wider nasal bridge, larger jaw, protruding chin, deeper voice and heavier brow ridge than females. Females have concluded a larger proportion of the soft tissue development of their nose by age 12, while the nose in males continues to grow to age 17 resulting in their having greater soft tissue dimensions of their nose.

Women in all ethnic populations tend to have lighter skin color than men. Women are more homogeneous in skin color than men. Elderly men are darker and redder in color than elderly women. Men are more likely to develop wrinkles than women and wrinkles are related to cumulative sun exposure. Hyperpigmentation, another photoaging parameter, is more common in women.

Males have thicker skin than females from age 5 to 90 years. Male skin progressively thins with advancing age but women maintain constant skin thickness until menopause, after which it progressively declines. Subcutaneous fat thickness is greater in women. The male forearm skin contains more collagen at all ages between 15–93 years. The ratio of collagen to thickness (collagen density) is lower in women. The rate of collagen loss is similar in men and women. Forearm skin fold thickness decreases starting at age 35 years for women and 45 years for men.

Dihydrotestosterone is responsible for terminal hair growth of the beard, chest, upper pubic triangle and external ears, sites of hair growth usually restricted to males. Levels of type II 5a-reductase are higher in males and higher in body areas affected by androgenetic alopecia. Women have about 1/3 the level of 5a-reductase as men. Females have higher cytochrome P-450 aromatase enzyme which is involved in converting androgens to estrogens within the hair follicle. Estrogen receptors have been identified in the skin, and females have a higher estrogen receptor content.

The distribution of fat over the body is different, with men tending to accumulate fat in the abdominal region and upper parts of the body and women in the lower body, particularly the gluteal and femoral regions. The proportion of body fat is higher in women than men. Females have lower glucocorticoid receptor density in the visceral preadipocytes than males. This difference may contribute to the smaller visceral fat mass in females. Lipoprotein lipase activity and mRNA levels are higher in women in the gluteal and abdominal regions. In women, higher enzyme activity is found in the gluteus rather than abdominal areas, while in men it is higher in the abdomen.

Age-related changes in the stratum corneum sphingolipid composition are found in women but not in men. Overall, males have higher sebum secretion rates. Sebum secretion is higher in males than females between ages 20 to 69 years but not from ages 15 to 19 years. In men between 50 to 70 years the sebum secretion output remains unaltered whereas in women in this age range the sebum output decreases.

From age 15–69 years, women exhibit longer blistering times than men in both antecubital and abdominal sites.

Women have a lower baseline transepidermal water loss as compared to men, but after irritation, similar values occur in both sexes. After hydration, cutaneous extensibility increases in women but not men. Changes in skin occur during the menstrual cycle. Transdermal water loss is higher on the day of minimal estrogen-progesterone secretion as compared to the day of maximal secretion.

Females in general have lower skin blood flow than males, but only after menarche and before menopause. During the menstrual cycle, finger blood flow decreases during the luteal phase compared with flow during the preovulatory phase. Women have decreased extremity blood flow owing to increased sympathetic outflow caused by estrogens. Basal hand blood flow, finger blood flow, and skin perfusion are greater in men than in women. Local cooling of the hand causes a greater decrease in cutaneous blood flow in females.

Skin circulation in females varies during the menstrual cycle. Basal flow is lowest in the luteal phase and highest in the preovulatory phase. Males have a higher basal cutaneous blood flow than young females, but not in women over age 50 years. Vasodilation due to local heating occurs at a lower skin temperature in females. Women tolerate cold better in the winter than men but no difference is found during the summer.

In response to musical stimulus, women have a greater decrease in finger temperature. When listening to tones, men exhibit more asymmetry in frequency and magnitude of skin conductance between hands with larger skin conductance response occurring on the left hand. In women, asymmetry was less marked and larger skin conductance response found on the right hand. These results suggest a possible cerebral hemispheric difference in response to auditory stimuli.

Women are more sensitive to small temperature changes and to pain caused by either heat or cold. The prickling pain threshold sensation provoked by heat projected to the skin from a lamp is lower in women. There are gender differences in current perception thresholds at 250 and 5 hertz.

Neonatal girls have a higher skin conductance than neonatal boys. Men sweat more than women. Histamine produces bigger wheals in women. Women have higher transcutaneous oxygen pressure values than men. In utero, boys appear to have delayed epidermal barrier maturation.

Trace elements in nails: Males have higher concentrations of iron and copper while women have higher concentrations of zinc in their nails. Women have been found to have higher metal content in their hair.

The female gingival smile line appears to be a female lineament and the low smile line seems to be a male lineament.

Diseases

Overall, females have a higher prevalence of skin pathology than males.

Abscess, Furuncle, and Carbuncle
    Male > Female

Acne
    Female > Male
    More severe in males.

Acne Aestivalis
    Female > Male

Acne Conglobata
    Male > Female

Acne Excorice des Jeunes Filles
    Female > Male

Acne Fulminans
    Male > Female
    It is primarily seen in teenage boys.

Acne Infantile
    Male > Female

Acne Keloidalis
    Male > Female
    It is primarily seen in black males.

Acne Roseacea
    Female > Male (3:1)
    Rhinophyma is more common in males (3:1). Females have 2 times more chin and cheek involvement.

Acne Vulgaris
    Male = Female
    Whites > Blacks, Asians
    It is more severe in males than females. Many women experience mild flares in connection with the increased progesterone released during the luteal phase of the menstrual cycle.

Acquired Hypertrichosis Lanuginosa
    Female > Male (3:1)

Acquired Total Lipodystrophy
    Female > Male

Acral Arteriovenous Hemangioma
    Male > Female

Acrochordon
    Female > Male

Acrogeria
    Female > Male

Acrokeratoelastoidosis of Costa
    Female > Male

Actinic Keratosis
    Male > Female
    It is primarily due to occupational sun exposure.

Actinic Prurigo
    Female > Male

Actinic Reticuloid
    Male > Female

Acute Intermittent Porphyria
    Female > Male (1.5–2:1)

Adiposis Dolorosa
    Female > Male

Adult T-Cell Leukemia/Lymphoma
    Male > Female

Ainhum
    Male > Female
    It is traditionally a disease of African males.
    Usually affects the 5th toe leading to amputation.

Alopecia
    Male > Female
    50% of white males have notable hair loss by age 50 years. In menopausal females, 37% show some hair loss.

Androgenetic Alopecia
    Male > Female

Angiocentric Lymphoma
    Male > Female

Angiokeratoma Circumscriptum
    Female > Male

Angiokeratoma Corporia Diffusum
    Male > Female

Angiokeratoma Fordyce
    Male > Female

Angiokeratoma of Mibelli
    Female > Male

Angioleiomyomas
    Female > Male

Angiolymphoid Hyperplasia with Eosinophilia
    Female > Male

Angioma Serpininosum
    Female > Male

Anosacral Cutaneous Amyloidosis
    Male > Female
    Primarily occurs in elderly Japanese males.

Apthous Stomatitis
    Female > Male

Apthous Ulcer
    Female > Male

Atheromatous Embolism
    Male > Female

Atherosclerosis Obliterans
    Male > Female

Atopic Dermatitis
    Male > Female (1.2:1)
    Females tend to have a worse prognosis. Females in one study had more allergic and irritant reactions to sunscreen products.

Atrophoderma of Pasini and Pierini
    Female > Male

Atypical Fibroxanthoma
    Male > Female

Atypical Pain Syndrome
    Female > Male

Autoerythrocyte Sensitization
    Female > Male
    Painful bruising occurs.

Baldness
    Male > Female

41% of men vs. 26% of women between 18–70 years of age have some degree of hair loss.

Males with androgenetic alopecia have hair loss that begins with bitemporal recession and thinning over the vertex. In contrast, women with androgenetic alopecia have diffuse thinning of the entire crown with retention of the frontal hairline. Also women do not develop the extent of hair loss because of higher levels of a protective aromatase enzyme that converts testosterone to estradiol.

Basal Cell Carcinoma
    Male > Female (2:1)
    It is the most common tumor of light-skinned people.
    Whites > Black, Nonasians
    It is more common in fair skinned blondes and redheads. Incidence is increasing in females due to lifestyle changes.
    It is uncommon in blacks.
    Risk increases with sunlight exposure.
    Risk of metastases is twice as high in males.
    More commonly seen on the ears in men and lower legs in women.

Basal Cell Nevus Syndrome
    Male = Female
    White > Black, Asian

Becker's Melanosis
    Female > Male (5:1)
    Often first noted after intense sun exposure.

Becker's Muscular Dystrophy
    Male > Female

Becker's Nevus
    Male > Female (2:1)

Behcet's Syndrome
    Male > Female (up to 2:1)
        In Western countries.
    Female prevalence higher in Korea and Japan.
    Asian > White
    Genital ulcers are painful in males, but are usually painless in females.

Erythema nodosum is common in females and usually occurs on the front of the legs.

Chronic progressive involvement of the central nervous system occurs in 10–20% of patients, particularly males in whom the disease begins at an early age.

Benign Angioendotheliomatosis
: Female > Male
It is especially noted in females who have subacute bacterial endocarditis.

Benign Cephalic Histiocytosis
: Male > Female (2:1)

Benign Mucus Membrane Pemphigoid
: Female > Male

Benign Symmetric Lipomatosis
: Male > Female
Usually alcoholics

Blastomycosis
: Male > Female (10:1)
The difference is probably due to occupational or environmental factors.

Bloom's Syndrome
: Male > Female (4:1)
Affected males tend to be infertile due to defective sperm.

Blue Nevus
: Female > Male (2:1)

Boweniod Papulosis (Viral Keratoses)
: Female > Male (slightly)
Cervical carcinoma in-situ in females seems to show a preferential association with HPV 16.

Bullous Pemphigoid
: Female > Male
Males tend to have more recalcitrant disease.
Antibodies to BP-180 are three times more common in males.

Buschke-Loewenstein Tumor
: Male > Female

Candida Onychomycosis
   Female > Male

Carbuncles and Furuncles
   Male > Female

Cat Scratch Disease
   Male > Female

Cellulitis
   Male = Female
   But perianal cellulitis is more common in boys.

Chancroid
   Male > Female

CHILD Syndrome
   Female > Male
   An ichythyosis form of dermatitis with congenital hemidysplasia and limb defects.

Chondrodermatitis Heliais
   Male > Female (9:1)

Chromoblastomycosis
   Male > Female

Chronic Actinic Dermatitis
   Female > Male (10:1)

Chronic Cutaneous Lupus Erythematosus
   Female > Male

Chronic Discoid Lupus Erythematosus
   Female > Male (2:1)

Chronic Urticaria/Angioedema
   Female > Male

Cicatricial Pemphigoid
   Female > Male (2:1)

Classic Porokeratosis (Mibelli)
   Male > Female (2–3:1)

Clear Cell Sarcoma
   Female > Male

Clubbing of Nails with Hypertrophic Osteooarthropathy
    Male > Female

Clubbing of Nails with Pachydermoperiostosis
    Male > Female

Coccidiodomycosis
    Male > Female

Cold Panniculitis
    Female > Male
        Adults
    Usually occurs on the thigh.

Contact Dermatitis
    Female > Male
    Black skin is less susceptible.
    Females have more positive patch test results.

Coumarin Necrosis of Skin
    Female > Male

Cryptococcosis
    Male > Female (3:1)

Cutaneous Angiosarcoma
    Male > Female

Cutaneous B-Cell Lymphoma
    Male > Female

Cutaneous Drug Reactions
    Female > Male (1.35:1)

Cutaneous Squamous Cell Carcinoma
    Male > Female

Cutaneous T-Cell Lymphoma
    Male > Female (2.7:1)

Cutaneous Tuberculosis
    Female > Male
        lupus vulgaris form
    Male > Female
        tuberculosis verrucosa cutis form

Cylindroma, Malignant
    Female > Male

Darier's Disease
    Male > Female

Delusions of Parasitosis (Ekbom's Disease)
    Female > Male (2:1)
        Overall
    Female = Male
        Less than age 50 years
    Female > Male (3:1)
        Over age 50 years

Dercum's Disease
    Female > Male

Dermatitis Artefacta
    Female > Male (3–8:1)

Dermatitis Herpetiformis
    Male > Female (1.5–2:1)

Dermatofibroma
    Female > Male

Dermatofibrosarcoma Protuberans
    Male > Female (4:1)

Dermatoheliosis
    Male > Female
    White > Black

Desmoid Tumor
    Female > Male

Desmoplastic Melanoma
    Female > Male
    White > Black

Desmoplastic Trichoepithelioma
    Female > Male

Digital Mucous Cyst
    Female > Male
    Usually occurs in middle age to elderly women.

Dissecting Cellulitis
   Male > Female
   Usually occurs in black men.
   It affects the vertex and occipital scalp.

Disseminated Cryptococcosis
   Male > Female (3:1)

Disseminated Gonococcal Infection
   Female > Male

Disseminated Superficial Actinic Porokeratosis
   Female > Male (3:1)

Donovanosis
   Male > Female

Duchenne Muscular Dystrophy
   Male > Female

Dupuytren's Contracture
   Male > Female (2–4:1)

Dyskeratosis Congenita
   Male > Female

Dysplastic Melanocytic Nevus
   Male = Female
   White > Black

Ehlers-Danlos Syndrome Types V and IX
   Male > Female

Elastofibroma Dorsi
   Female > Male

Elastosis Perforans Serpiginosa
   Male > Female (4:1)

Endemic Kaposi's Sarcoma — African
   Male > Female (3–10:1)
      Children
   Male > Female (18:1)
      Adults
   Earlier onset in adult female with more rapid generalization in females.

Eosinophilic Fasciitis
   Male > Female (3:1)

Epidermal Inclusion Cyst
   Male > Female

Erosive Pustular Dermatosis
   Females only
   Restricted to scalp of females > 70 years old.

Erysipeloid
   Male > Female (3:1)

Erythema Infectiosum
   Female > Male
       Symptomatic illness

Erythemalgia
   Male > Female (11:3)

Erythema Multiforma Minor
   Female > Male (slightly)

Erythema Multiforme
   Male > Female (3:2)

Erythema Nodosum
   Female > Male (3–4:1)

Erythema Paranasale
   Male > Female

Erythrasma
   Male > Female

Erythrocyanosis
   Female > Male

Erythroplasia
   Male > Female
   In males, frequently seen on the floor of the mouth, whereas in women, the tongue and buccal mucosa are more involved.

Erythroplasia of Queyrat
   Male > Female

Exfoliative Dermatitis
  Male > Female (2–3:1)

Exfoliative Erythroderma Syndrome
  Male > Female

Extramammary Paget's Disease
  Female > Male

Fabry's Disease
  Male > Female

Factitious Syndrome
  Female > Male

Focal Dermal Hypoplasia
  Female > Male (9:1)

Follicular Degeneration Syndrome
  Female > Male

Folliculitis
  Male > Female

Fox-Fordyce Disease
  Female > Male (9–10:1)

Generalized Essential Telangiectasia
  Female > Male

Generalized Lipodystrophy
  Female > Male

Giant Cell Arteritis
  Female > Male (2:1)

Glomus Tumor
  Female > Male
  Subungual Glomus Tumor: Female > Male (3:1)

Goltz's Syndrome
  Female only
  X-linked dominant and tends to be lethal to male embryos.

Gonorrhea
  Male > Female
    Symptomatic infection

Gout
> Male > Female (95% of cases in males)
> Females have mean serum urate levels 1 mg/dl lower than men until after menopause. This may explain the sex difference.

Granular Cell Tumor
> Female > Male

Granuloma Annulare
> Female > Male (2:1)

Granuloma Faciale
> Male > Female

Granulomatous Slack Skin
> Female > Male

Graves' Disease
> Female > Male

Grover's Disease
> Male > Female

Halo Nevomelanocytic Nevus
> Male > Female (2:1)

Hemangioma, Congenital
> Female > Male (3:1)

Hereditary Coproporphyria
> Female > Male

Hereditary Polymorphic Light Eruption of Native Americans
> Female > Male (2:1)

Herpes Gladiatorum
> Male > Female

Herpes Simplex Genital Infection
> Female > Male

Hidradenitis Suppurativa
> Female > Male
> But females tend to develop axillary form and males develop perianal form.

Hidroadenoma Papilliferum
  Female > Male

Hirsutism
  Female > Male
  Whites > Blacks > Asians

HIV
  Male > Female
    In the United States.

Hoigne Syndrome
  Male > Female
  A psuedoanaphylactic reaction to procaine penicillin injection.

Hori's Nevus
  Female > Male
  Primarily in Japanese women.

Hunter Syndrome
  Male > Female

Hypereosinophilic Syndrome
  Male > Female

Hypergammaglobulinemic Purpura
  Female > Male

Hyperkeratotic Palmar Eczema
  Male > Female

Hypohidrotic Ectodermal Dysplasia
  Male > Female

Hypomelanosis of Ito
  Female > Male (2.5:1)

Hypothyroidism
  Female > Male

Ichthyosis Nigricans
  Males only
  X-linked disorder, female carriers may show partial abnormalities.

Idiopathic Hirsutism
  Female > Male

Idiopathic Toxic Epidermal Necrolysis
   Female > Male

Incontinentia Pigmenti
   Female > Male
   97% are females, lethal in males.

Infantile Acropustulosis
   Male > Female
   It primarily occurs in blacks.

Intraepidermal Epithelioma
   Male > Female
   Primarily seen in white middle aged men.

Irritant Contact Dermatitis
   Female > Male
   People with fair skin are more prone to ICD.

Kaposi's Sarcoma, Classic
   Male > Female (15:1)
   Primarily affects elderly men of Eastern European and Mediterranean origin.

Kaposi's Sarcoma, Immunosupression Associated
   Male > Female (2–4:1)
   Highest incidence in homosexual men. AIDS-related Kaposi's sarcoma affects > 35% of AIDS cases.

Kawasaki Disease
   Male > Female (1.5:1)

Keloids
   Male = Female
   Black > White

Keratoacanthoma
   Male > Female (2:1)
   Whites > Blacks, Asians

Keratoderma Climacterium
   Female > Male

Keratosis Follicularis Spinulosa Decalvans
   Males have more severe disease.

Ketinic Reticuloid
    Female > Male

Kimura's Disease
    Male > Female
    Primarily seen in Asians.

Kinky Hair Disease
    Female only
    Lethal in male embryos.

Kyrle's Disease
    Female > Male (2:1)

Langerhans Cell Histiocytosis
    Male > Female (2:1)

Large Plaque Parapsoriasis
    Male > Female
    Breast frequently involved in females.

Latex Allergy
    Male > Female (2:1)
    General population, excluding health care workers.
    As more females work in health care industry, the ratio may be different in this population.

Leiomyomas
    Female > Male

Leiomyosarcoma
    Male > Female

Lentigo Maligna
    Male = Female
    White > Black

Leprosy
    Male > Female
    Blacks have less severe disease.

Leukodermal Punctatum
    Female > Male

Leukoplakia
    Male > Female (slightly)

Lichen Nitidus
    Female > Male
    Generalized Eruption

Lichen Planus
    Female > Male
    Hypertrophic LP more common in blacks.

Lichen Sclerosis et Atrophicus
    Female > Male (10:1)
    Primarily menopausal women.

Lichen Simplex Chronicus
    Female > Male
    Asian, Nonasian > Whites

Lichen Spinulisus
    Female > Male

Lichen Striatus
    Female > Male (2–3:1)

Linear IgA Bullous Disease of Childhood
    Female > Male (3:2)

Lipedematous Alopecia
    Females only

Livedo Reticularis
    Female > Male

Livedoid Vasculitis
    Female > Male

Lobular Panniculitis Associated with Pancreatic Disease
    Male > Female (5:1)
        Associated with pancreatic cancer
    Male > Female (3:1)
        Associated with pancreatitis, 65% are chronic alcoholics.

Localized Heat Urticaria
    Female > Male

Localized Scleroderma
    Female > Male (3:1)

Loose Anagen Syndrome
    Female > Male

Lupus Erythematosus Profundus
    Female > Male

Lupus Panniculitis
    Female > Male

Lupus Pernio
    Female > Male

Lupus Vulgaris (Cutaneous Tuberculosis)
    Female > Male (2–3:1)

Lymphadenosis Benigna Cutis
    Female > Male

Lymphangioma Circumscriptum
    Female > Male

Lymphedema
    Female > Male (3.5:1)
    Especially lymphedema praecox

Lymphogranuloma Venereum
    Male > Female (5:1)

Macular Amyloidosis
    Female > Male

Malignant Atrophic Papulosis
    Male > Female (3:2)

Mammary Paget's Disease
    Female > Male

Mastitis/Abscess of Infant Breast
    Female > Male (2:1)

Melanocytic Nevocellular Nevi
    Male = Female
    Whites > Blacks

Melanoma
    Male > Female (slightly)

Males are more likely to develop melanoma on the anterior torso and midback, females on the lower legs, especially the posterior calves. Midback lesions carry worse prognosis.
Under age 40, more common in females but > age 45, more common in males.
Females survive longer than males.
Superficial spreading melanoma most frequently involves the trunk and back in males and lower extremities in females. In nodular melanoma, most common site is trunk in males and legs in females.
Males are more likely to develop melanoma of the ears.
Increasingly found on the trunk in both sexes.
Rates are increasing in both sexes.
Thin melanomas in women have a higher expression of melanoma associated antigen G7-E2 while men have higher expression of the histocompatibility antigen HLA-DR.

Melasma
Female > Male (9:1)
1/3 of cases in females and most cases in males are idiopathic.
Asian, Hispanic > White

Menkes' Kinky Hair Syndrome
Male > Female

Menkes' Steely Hair Disease
Male > Female

Metastatic Melanoma with Unknown Primary
Male > Female (3:1)

Molluscum Contagiosum
Male > Female

Mongolian Spot
Male = Female
Asian, Nonasian > Blacks > Whites

Morphea
Female > Male (3:1)

Mucocele
Male > Female

Multicentric Reticulohistiocytosis
　　Female > Male

Multiple Lentigines Syndrome
　　Male > Female

Multiple Miliary Osteoma of the Face
　　Female > Male

Multiple Miliary Osteomas of the Face and Scalp, Late Onset
　　Female > Male

Mycetoma
　　Male > Female (9:1)

Mycobacterium Fortuitum Complex
　　Female > Male

Mycobacterium Marinum
　　Male > Female

Mycobacterium Ulcerans
　　Female > Male

Mycoses Fungoides
　　Male > Female (2:1)

Nasal Lentiginous Melanoma
　　Male > Female (3:1)
　　White > Blacks, Asians
　　Principal melanoma in blacks.

Necrobiosis Lipoidica Diabeticorum
　　Female > Male (3:1)

Nerve Sheath Myxoma
　　Female > Male

Neurodermatitis
　　Female > Male
　　Nucchal and suboccipital area more affected in women, perianal area more affected in males.

Neurofibromatosis
　　Male > Female (slightly)

Neurotic Excoriations
    Female > Male

Nevus Anemicus
    Female > Male

Nevus of Ota
    Female > Male (5:1)
    Asian > Blacks > Whites

Nickel Dermatitis
    Female > Male (10:1)

Nodular Melanoma
    Male = Female
    White > Black

Nodular Vasculitis
    Female > Male

Nummular Eczema
    Male > Female
    Females have 2 peaks of onset—age 15–25 years and 55–65 years. Males peak age is at 55–65 years.

Occupational Hand Irritant Dermatitis
    Female > Male

Onychomycosis
    Female > Male
    Toenail infection is 4–6 times more common than fingernail infection.

Oraficial Tuberculosis
    Male > Female

Oral Candidiasis
    Female > Male

Oral Hairy Leukoplakia
    Male > Female

Oral Leukoplakia
    Male > Female (2:1)

Oral Lichen Planus
    Females are more symptomatic.
Oral Nevi
    Female > Male (slightly)
Oral Squamous Acanthosis
    Male > Female
Paget's Disease
    Female > Male
Palmoplantar Pustulosis
    Female > Male (4:1)
Pancreatic Panniculitis
    Male > Female
Papular Xanthomas
    Male > Female
Paronychia
    Female > Male (9:1)
        Chronic
    Male = Female
        Acute
Partial Lipodystrophy
    Female > Male (4:1)
Pediculosis
    Female > Male
Pediculosis Captitis
    Female > Male
Pediculosis Pubis
    Male > Female
Pemphigoid, Bullous
    Female > Male
Perioral Dermatitis
    Female > Male
PHACES Syndrome
    Female > Male (9:1)

Primarily female infants. They have hemangiomas of the cervico-facial region.

Piezogenic Papules
    Female > Male

Pigmented Hairy Nevus (Becker)
    Male > Female

Pigmented Peribuccal Erythema of Brocq
    Female > Male

Pigmented Purpuric Dermatosis
    Male > Female

Pilomatrixoma
    Female > Male

Pilonidal Disease
    Male > Female (2.2:1)

Pitted Keratolysis
    Male > Female

Pityriasis Lichenoides Chronica
    Male > Female

Pityriasis Lichenoides et Varioliformis
    Male > Female

Pityriasis Rosea
    Female > Male (1.5:1)

Plantar Bromhidrosis
    Male > Female

Plummer-Vinson Syndrome
    Female > Male

Polyarteritis Nodosa
    Male > Female (2.5:1)
        Adult
    Male = Female
        Pediatric

Polymorphic Light Eruption
   Female > Male (2–3:1)
   Nonasians have hereditary variety.

Pomade Acne
   Male > Female
   Primarily seen in blacks.

Porokeratosis of Mibelli
   Male > Female (2:1)

Porokeratosis Plantaris, Palmaris et Disseminata
   Male > Female (2:1)

Porphyria Cutanea Tarda
   Male > Female
   Prevalence increases in females with use of oral contraceptives.

Postphlebitic Syndrome
   Female > Male

Primary and Myeloma-Associated Systemic Amyloidosis
   Male > Female (slightly)
   Mucocutaneous involvement occurs in 40%.

Primary Raynaud's Disease
   Female > Male (4:1)

Proliferating Trichilemmal Cyst
   Female > Male (4:1)

Proliferating Trichilemmal Tumor
   Female > Male
   Primarily in elderly women.

Pseudofolliculitis Barbae
   Male > Female
   Primarily in black males.

Pseudolymphoma
   Female > Male

Psoriasis
   Female = Male
   Two peaks in age of onset of nonpustular psoriais—at age 16 years in females and 22 years in males and age 60 years in both sexes.

Whites > Blacks, Nonasians, Asians
Different HLA gene associations have been shown in male and female patients.
Smoking may be a risk factor for psoriasis onset, especially in women.
Psoriasis in the diaper area is more common in female infants.

Psoriasis Vulgaris, Erythrodermic
    Male > Female

Pustular Palmoplantar Psoriasis
    Female > Male (3:1)

Pyoderma Faciale
    Female > Male
    Primarily postadolescent females.

Pyogenic Granuloma
    Female > Male (slightly)

Raynaud's Disease/Phenomenon
    Female > Male

Reiter's Syndrome
    Male > Female (9:1)
        Endemic or venereal form
    Male = Female
        Epidemic or postdysenteric form

Rhabdomyoma
    Male > Female
        Adult type
        Usually in muscle of mucosa head
    Male > Female
        Fetal type
        Usually involves ear
    Female > Male
        Genital type

Rheumatoid Arthritis
    Female > Male

Vasculitis is more common in females.

Arteritic ulcers are more common in females with nodules and who are positive for ANA and Rheumatoid Factor.

Transparent skin more commonly seen in females, and increases with age.

Riehl's Melanosis
  Female > Male

Rosacea
  Female > Male (3:1)
  Whites > Blacks
  Males tend to have more severe disease.
  Rhinophyma occurs more in males.
  Females more likely to develop symptoms on the cheeks (87% vs. 68%) while men more likely to develop severe symptoms on the nose (21% vs. 8%).

Rosacea Conglobata
  Female > Male

Rosacea Fulminans
  Female > Male
  Primarily in young women.

Rothmund-Thomson Syndrome
  Male > Female (2:1)

Rud's Syndrome
  Male > Female

Sarcoidosis Leukoderma
  Female > Male

Scleroderma
  Female > Male (4:1)

Sebaceous Gland Cancer
  Female > Male

Seborrheic Dermatitis
  Male > Female (slightly)

Seborrheic Keratoses
  Male > Female

Sezary Syndrome
    Male > Female

Sjogren's Syndrome
    Female > Male
    Mothers with Sjogren's may passively transfer antiplatelet antibodies to their neonates and induce ITP.

Skin Tag
    Female > Male

Small Plaque Parapsoriasis
    Male > Female (3:1)

Solar Keratosis
    Male > Female
    White > Black

Solar Lentigo
    Male = Female
    White > Asian > Black

Solar Urticaria
    Female > Male (3:1)

Spider Angioma
    Female > Male

Spindle Cell Hemangioendothelioma
    Male > Female

Spindle Cell Lipoma
    Male > Female

Sporotrichosis
    Male > Female

Spotted Fevers
    Male > Female

Squamous Cell Carcinoma
    Male > Female (2–3:1)
    White > Black

More frequent on legs of females.
Rates increase with age and sun exposure.
4 times less common than basal cell carcinoma in the U.S.
Body distribution difference noted among races and less frequent in blacks.
Rates increasing in both sexes.

Stasis Dermatitis
Female > Male

Stevens-Johnson Syndrome
Male > Female (2:1)

Still's Disease
Female > Male
Polyarticular type
Female = Male
Pauciarticular type
Early onset in females—often have chronic iridocyclitis
Late onset in males—often involves large joints of lower leg and spine.
Rash occurs in 25% of boys.

Striae
Female > Male
70% of adolescent females and 40% of adolescent males develop striae.

Subacute Cutaneous Lupus Erythematosus
Female > Male
White > Black, Hispanic

Subacute Nodular Migratory Panniculitis
Female > Male

Subcorneal Pustular Dermatosis
Female > Male

Subungual Exostoses
Female > Male
Usually on great toe.

Sunburn
    Male = Female
    White > Blacks, Asian, Hispanics

Superficial Spreading Melanoma
    Female > Male

Sweet's Syndrome
    Female > Male
            Idiopathic form
    Female = Male
            Associated with hematologic disorder

Syphilis
    Male > Female (2–4:1)

Syringoma
    Female > Male

Systemic Lupus Erythematosus
    Female > Male (8:1)
    Black > White
    Males tend to present more often with atypical skin manifestations including widespread discoid lupus erythematosus and papular and nodular mucinosis.

Systemic Scleroderma
    Female > Male (4:1)

T-cell Immunoblastic Lymphoma
    Male > Female

Takayasu's Arteritis
    Female > Male (8:1)

Telogen Effluvium
    Female > Male

Thromboangiitis Obliterans
    Male > Female
    Primarily in tobacco smokers, especially of Asian descent.

Tinea Barbae
    Males only

Tinea Capitis
    Males > Female (5:1)

Tinea Cruris
    Male > Female

Tinea Pedis
    Male > Female

Tinea Unguium
    Male > Female

Toxic Shock Syndrome
    Female > Male
    Usually in menstruating women.

Transient Acantholytic Dermatosis (Grover's Disease)
    Male > Female

Trichilemmal Cyst
    Female > Male

Trichotillomania
    Female > Male (5:1)

Tuberculosis Verrucous Cutis
    Male > Female

Tularemia
    Male > Female

Unilateral Nevoid Telangiectasia
    Male > Female
        Congenital form
    Female > Male
        Acquired form—appears at puberty with rise in estrogen levels

Urticaria
    Male = Female
    But chronic urticaria more common in middle age to older females.

Urticarial Vasculitis
    Female > Male (3:1)

Varicose Veins
    Female > Male (3:1)

Variegate Porphyria
    Male = Female
    But females have more frequent attacks typical of acute intermittent porphyria and males are more likely to have the skin lesions of porphyria cutanea tarda.

Venous Leg Ulcers
    Female > Male

Verruca Plana
    Female > Male

Verruca Plantaris
    Female > Male

Verruca Vulgaris
    Male > Female (slightly)

Verrucous Carcinoma of the Skin
    Male > Female (4.5:1)

Warfarin Necrosis
    Female > Male

Warts
    Female > Male

Warts, Plantar
    Female > Male (slightly)

Weber-Christian Disease
    Female > Male

Wegener's Granulomatosus
    Male > Female (1.3–3:1–2)
    Skin disease occurs in 40–50% of cases.
    White > Black

Wrinkling of Skin
    Men notice wrinkles about 10 years later than women. About 85% of face lifts are in women.
    Women's skin is thinner and drier, whereas men's faces have thicker skin and more active oil glands.

Women more susceptible to wrinkling effects of smoking than men. The relative risk of wrinkling from smoking is 2.3 in men and 3.1 in women.

Xanthoma Disseminatum
    Male > Female

X-linked Ichthyosis
    Female > Male

X-linked Ocular Albinism of Nettleship-Falls
    Male > Females
    Found in Amish families

X-linked Ocular Albinism with Sensorineural Deafness
    Male > Female

Zipkowski-Margolis Syndrome
    Male > Female

Neurology

Anatomy and Physiology

The adult brain weighs 1050–1550 grams (average 1275 grams) in females and 1100–1700 grams (average 1400 grams) in males. The ventricular size and sulcal size are larger in males.

Several formulae have been constructed to give cranial capacity from the length, breadth and height of the cranium. Examples are:

Males: 0.000337 (L-11) (B-11) (H-11) + 406.01 cc
Females: 0.000400 (L-11) (B-11) (H-11) + 206.6 cc

The thickness of the calvaria in Caucasians (from 15 to 82 years) averages 5.8 mm. In males, thickness increases with age, in females the reverse is true. There is little sexual difference in skulls until puberty; the adult female's is a little lighter and smaller, its capacity about 10% less; its walls are thinner and muscular ridges less marked; the glabella, superciliary arches and mastoid processes are less prominent; air sinuses are smaller; tympanic plates are smaller and their margins less rough; the upper orbital margins are sharper, the forehead vertical, the frontal and parietal tuberosities prominent and the vault somewhat flattened; the facial contour is rounder, facial bones smoother and the mandible and maxillae and contained teeth are smaller. The skull is thinner in women and children

The brain volume is about 91 ml higher in men and the CSF volume is 20 ml higher in men. Females have smaller cerebellar volume than males of the same age (122 ± 16 ml in males versus 104 ± 10 ml in females). White matter signal intensity of the brain on magnetic resonance imaging is higher in females.

Differences in the size and symmetry of the temporal lobes, corpus callosum and various hypothalmic nuclei such as the suprachiasmatic nucleus, the sexually dimorphic nucleus, and the interstitial nucleus of the anterior hypothalamus have been reported between males and females. The corpus callosum is overall larger in males but the isthmus and splenium of the corpus callosum appear larger in females. The splenium is more bulbous shaped in females and more tubular shaped in males. The sexually dimorphic nuclei are twice as large in the adult male as in the adult female. The suprachiasmatic nucleus is elongated in females and more spherical in males. The pituitary gland has a more convex upper margin in females. Males show an asymmetric pattern of increased fissurization of the left anterior cingulate, while females show greater symmetry with less fissurization of the left anterior cingulate.

Cerebral maturation may be more rapid in girls as are physical and psychological development. Male newborns have significantly larger head/chest proportions, suggesting they may have a greater metabolic demand, related to brain size. During brain development of children and adolescents, males have more prominent age-related gray matter decrease and white matter volume and corpus callosal area increase compared to females. In children under age 9 years, the amygdala appears to be more active in males than that of adults or female children.

Women have higher rates of cerebral blood flow until the sixth decade when flow rates are similar. Blood velocity in the middle cerebral artery is higher in females up to age 50 years.

Sexual dimorphism of thoracolumbar vertebrae has been observed, with female vertebral bodies being more slender from the eighth year onwards: there being greater growth in transverse diameter in males. The spinal canal has a gradual decrease in measurement between L1 and L5, with a greater relative width in the female. Female vertebral bodies have a lower ratio of width to depth. Males have a higher fat concentration in the lumbar vertebra.

Brain atrophy in elderly men affects primarily the left hemisphere, whereas it is more symmetric in elderly females. An activation of vasopressinergic neurons is found during ageing in the supraoptic nucleus in females but not males. Age-related shrinkage of the putamen and caudate nucleus are seen in males more so than females. The APOE epsilon 4 allele is associated with normal age-related cognitive decline in elderly females. Axons in the lateral corticospinal tract decrease in area and diameter with ageing in males but not in females.

The amplitude of the sensory action potential recorded at midcalf is 32% higher in females than in males. Somatosensory evoked potentials showed greater P40-N50 amplitude in females after posterior tibial nerve stimulation

Women show more right-sided serotonergic binding sites than men. Males synthesize serotonin at a 52% higher rate than females. Men and women have different rates of resting glucose metabolism of the limbic system and this is felt to be associated with gender differences in thought and emotional processing. Adult males have 10–30% higher butylcholinesterase activity than adult females.

Estradiol levels are associated with 5-HT (5-hydroxytryptamine) levels in the brain. With high estradiol, the level of 5-HT also increases in the brain. Estrogen increases the efficacy of synapses and long-term potentiation and potentiates neuronal transmission in the hippocampus. Estrogen also augments cerebral blood flow, cholinergic function, and cerebral glucose metabolism. The amount of estrogen appears to decrease in brains of adult females postmenopausally but elderly males maintain a high level of estrogen in their brains as they age.

Cortical glucose metabolism is 19% greater in premenopausal females than age-matched males. Concentrations of several neurotransmitter metabolites (choline. glutamate, glutamine, GABA, inositol, N-acetyl aspartate, glucose and lactate) are greater in the orbital frontal cortex (2%) and sensorimotor cortex (9%) in women compared to men. Females have lower dopamine (DA) but higher 3, 4-dihydroxyphenylacetic acid (DOPAC) levels and a higher DOPAC/DA ratio than males in the putamen. Dopamine D2-like receptor binding potentials in the frontal cortex, temporal cortex and thalamus are higher in females, especially in the frontal cortex. Males and females have differences in the muscarinic acetylcholinergic receptors in the brain. Males have fewer peaks of chromogranin A release per 8 hours than females. Females have more prolactin receptors in the choroid plexus than men. The orbital frontal cortex (OFC) in men has decreased chemical concentration compared to women, especially of N-acetyl aspartate. Males show larger effects of anxiety on OFC chemistry.

Males tend to show more accentuated cortical asymmetry and stronger right hemispheric dominance compared to females. Females typically show more diffuse lateralization patterns and greater left hemispheric bias than males. Females and males use different parts of their brains when performing certain tasks. On verbal tasks, males use primarily the left frontal hemisphere whereas females use their bifrontal hemispheres. Women tend to have more bilateral organization of brain function for many cognitive skills including language and visual recognition of faces. Females use the posterior temporal lobes more bilaterally during linguistic processing of global structures in a narrative than men do. In a recent study by fMRI to study brain organization during performance of a navigational skill, males activated the left hippocampus but females activated the right parietal cortex and right prefrontal cortex during the same task.

Female infants babble more and possess a larger vocabulary than male infants. Males and females exhibit different patterns of brain activation during phonological processing. Girls acquire articulatory facility somewhat earlier than boys. Male infants' sleeping rhythm seems to develop later than female infants and male infants sleep for shorter periods at night.

Females have greater manual dexterity and flexibility than males. Females excel in verbal skills and males in mathematical and visuo-spatial tasks. Females rely on both sides of the brain for certain aspects of language while men primarily rely on the left hemisphere.

Women show stronger right-handedness and better verbal skills than men. Hand preference is correlated with the anatomy of the sylvian fissure in men but not in women.

Gait: Female steps are quicker and shorter and movement of the trunk and hips is more graceful and delicate than males.

Smell: Females have more acute sense of smell. The olfactory activity in females varies throughout the menstrual cycle.

During negative affect (sadness) males show brain activity in the amygdala but not females. There is a suggestion of more focal and subcortical processing of sadness in men. Enhanced activity of the right amygdala in men is related to emotionally enhanced memory. Conversely, enhanced activity of the left amygdala in women is related to emotionally enhanced memory.

Pain threshold and tolerance to pain is lower in females. Females show greater sensitivity than men to noxious stimuli—more consistently to electrical, mechanical, ischemic and cold pressure than to thermal stimuli. Women are more likely to show a summation effect, a progressively increased response to repeated stimuli.

The period of freerunning circadian rhythms is shorter, and the fraction of sleep is larger in females than in males as long as the rhythms run internally synchronized.

Diseases

Abdominal Migraine
    Female > Male

Absence Seizure Disorder
    Female > Male (2:1)

Acquired Epileptic Aphasia
    Male > Female (2:1)

Acroparesthesias
    Female > Male

Adie Syndrome
    Female > Male

Adrenoleukodystrophy
    Male > Female

Alcoholic Myopathy
    Female > Male
    Females have lower gastric alcohol dehydrogenase and may metabolize alcohol slower.

Alcoholic Neuropathy
    Male > Female
    But females may be more susceptible to lower doses than males.

Alzheimer's Disease
    Female > Male (1.5:1)
    Unilateral left hemispheric defects are more common in women.
    Cognitive decline is more severe and accelerated in females, yet males have a higher mortality rate (probably due to comorbid conditions). Age adjusted death rate is 2.6 per 100,000 in men and 2.8 in women.
    Females have more unilateral left hemisphere perfusion defects on SPECT scans.
    Women with AD have more heterogenity in regional cerebral blood flow.
    Women with AD tend to perform worse than males with AD on tests of naming, verbal fluency, delayed word recall, constructional praxis and the general cognition score on AD Assessment Scale tests.

Aggressive behavior is seen more in males with AD.

Males are more likely to be apathetic and exhibit pacing, whereas women are more likely to be depressed, hoard, and be emotionally labile and psychotic. Women with AD are 2–4 times more likely to be depressed as men with AD.

In some studies, phosphorous metabolism in the frontal lobes was reduced in female patients compared to male patients.

Males with Down's Syndrome seem more likely to develop AD than females with Down's syndrome.

Women who develop AD early in life have less frontal function than men; such difference is not seen in women with late-onset AD.

Amyotrophic Lateral Sclerosis
Male > Female (1.3–3:1–2)
Females tend to live slightly longer than males with ALS.
Bulbar presentation is more common in older females.

Anencephaly
Female > Male (3–7:1)

Aphasia
After anterior damage to the brain, women incur aphasia more often than men (65% vs. 29%). In men, posterior damage more often affects speech (60% vs. 12%). Men develop aphasia more often from left hemisphere damage than women do. Men rely more on this hemisphere for speech than women.

Apraxia
Men are more likely to experience apraxia from left posterior damage than do women.

Arteriovenous Malformation
Females have a higher proportion of left hemisphere AVMs whereas males show an opposite trend.

Asperger's Disorder
Male > Female (4:1)

Atypical Facial Pain
Female > Male

Atypical Odontalgia
Female > Male

Autism
    Male > Female (3.8:1)

Behcet's Syndrome
    Male > Female

Bell's Palsy
    Female > Male (2–4:1)
        Overall
    Pregnant female has a 3.3 time greater risk of illness than non-pregnant female.
    Female > Male (2:1)
        Age 10–19 years
    Male = Female
        Age 20–40 years
    Female > Male (1.5:1)
        Age > 40 years

Blepharoclonus and Blepharospasm
    Female > Male

Bloch-Sulzberger Syndrome
    Females only

Brachial Neuritis
    Male > Female (2.4:1)

Brachial Plexus Neuropathy
    Male > Female

Brachycephaly
    Male > Female

Brain Abscess
    Male > Female (2:1)

Brain Injury, Traumatic
    Male > Female

Brain Neoplasm
    Male > Female (9:8)
    Predominant age is > 75 years in men, 65–74 years in women.

Brain Tumors
   Male > Female (slightly)
   More frequent in males than females in infancy and early childhood.

Briquet Disease
   Female > Male

Burning Tongue
   Female > Male

Call-Fleming Syndrome
   Female > Male

Carnitine Palmitoyl Transferase II Deficiency
   Female > Male

Carotid-Cavernous Sinus Fistula—Dural Type
   Female > Male

Carotid Stenosis
   Male > Female (3.8:2.7)
   Women have less severe disease; however restenosis after carotid endarterectomy is more common among women than men.
   Women are more likely to have carotid bruits.
   For each 10% increase in stenosis, the risk of stroke increases 26%.

Carotidynia
   Female > Male

Central Sleep Apnea
   Male > Female

Cerebellar Degeneration in Alcoholism
   Male > Female

Cerebral Palsy
   Male > Female (1.3:1)

Cervical Dystonia
   Female > Male (3–3.6:1–2)

Cervical Spine Injuries
   Male > Female (3:2)
   Males more likely to be involved in high speed motor vehicle wrecks and play more contact sports.

Cervical Spondylosis
  Male > Female (slightly)
  At age 59 years—70% of females and 85% of males have x-ray changes.
  At age 70 years—93% of females and 97% males have x-ray findings.

Cervical Strain
  In athletes, cervical strain injuries are more common in females.

Cervicogenic Headache
  Female > Male

Charcot-Marie Tooth Disease
  Male > Female (3:1)

Chordoma
  Male > Female (5:3)
  Females are more likely to have cranial presentation.

Choroideremia
  Male > Female

Chronic Headache
  Female > Male
  The lifetime prevalence of migraine is 25% in women and 8% in men, whereas it is 88% in females and 69% in males for tension-type headache.
  Boys begin to experience migraines earlier than girls with a peak age of onset of 5 years in boys and age 12 years in girls. After age 11 years more girls have migraines.
  Migraines persist for more years in girls and by age 25 years, migraines will resolve for 33% of men but only 15% for women who report childhood migraines.
  Spontaneous menopause is associated with improvement in migraines but worsening in tension-type headaches (67% of migraines improve but 60% of tension-type headaches worsen).
  Women are 1.6 times more likely to report unilateral headache and 2 times more likely to report nausea or visual symptoms.
  Exercise is more likely to be a headache trigger in men.
  Women more likely to identify foods as a headache trigger.

Men are more likely to report headache-related disability.
Cycling of estradiol, as during menses, is often associated with worse headache.

Chronic Inflammatory Demyelinating Polyradiculoneuropathy
Male > Female (slightly)

Chronic Paroxysmal Hemicrania
Female > Male (7:1)

Chronic Tension Headache
Female > Male
Exercise is reported as a more frequent trigger in men, and foods are identified as a more frequent trigger in women.

Cluster Headache
Male > Female (6–10:1)

Concussion
Male > Female (2:1)

Congenital Hydrocephalus
Male > Female

Congenital Inarticulation
Male > Female

Craniostenoses
Male > Female

Dissection of the Internal Carotid Artery
Female > Male
Primarily occurs in adult females in their 30–40's years of age.

Dyslexia
Male > Female (1.1–1.8:1)

Dystrophinopathies
Male > Female

Emery-Dreifuss Muscular Dystrophy
Male > Female
Disease is worse in males. Can develop cardiac conduction problems.

Empty-Sella Syndrome
Female > Male

Eosinophilic Myositis
  Male > Female

Ependymoma of the Fourth Ventricle
  Male > Female (2:1)

Epilepsy
  Male > Female
  In one series, women with temporal lobe epilepsy had 38% more endocrine disorders. Women with generalized epilepsy are also more prone to endocrine disorders.
  Men with temporal lobe epilepsy have more brain atrophy and are more vulnerable to seizure-associated brain abnormalities than are women.
  Epilepsy is more common in males in infancy.
  2/3rds of men and 50% of women with epilepsy have sexual dysfunction.

Exertional Headache
  Male > Female

Fabry's Disease
  Male > Female

Febrile Seizures
  Male > Female (slightly)

Fibromuscular Dysplasia of Blood Vessels
  Female > Male

Focal Dermal Hypoplasia
  Females only

Fragile-X Syndrome
  Male > Female (2:1)
  Males are usually more severely affected (80% will have moderate to severe retardation), only one third of females are retarded. 1 in 1250 males are affected and 1 in 5000 are transmitting males. 1 in 2000 females are affected and 1 in 700 females are carriers.

Garcis-Mason Syndrome
  Male > Female

Glioblastoma Multiforme
  Male > Female (2:1)

Glioma of the Optic Nerve and Chiasm
    Female > Male (2:1)

Glomus Jugulare Tumor
    Female > Male

Granulomatous Angiitis of the Central Nervous System
    Male > Female (slightly)

Guillain-Barre Syndrome
    Male > Female (1.5:1)

Headache and Psychiatric Disorders in Children
    Among girls, headaches are associated with depression and anxiety disorders.
    Among boys, headaches are associated with conduct disorders.

Hemicrania Continua
    Female > Male

Hemifacial Spasm
    Female > Male (2:1)

Hemophilus Influenza Meningitis
    Male > Female

Hippocampal Malrotation with Normal Corpus Callosum
    Male > Female

Hydrocephalus due to Stenosis of Aqueduct of Sylvius
    Male > Female

Hypokalemic Periodic Paralysis
    Male > Female (3–4:1)

Hypnic Headache
    Female > Male

Idiopathic Intracranial Hypertension
    Female > Male
    19 fold increase in young obese women.

Inclusion Body Myositis
    Male > Female (4:1)

Infantile Spasms
    Male > Female

Insomnia
    Female > Male

Juvenile Proximal Muscular Atrophy
    Male > Female

Kallmann Syndrome
    Male > Female

Kennedy Disease
    Male > Female

Klein-Levin Syndrome
    Male > Female

Lambert—Eaton Myasthenic Syndrome
    Male > Female (2–5:1)

Language Disorders
    Male > Female
    85% of affected children are males.

Leber's Hereditary Optic Neuropathy
    Male > Female

Lesch-Nyhan Syndrome
    Male > Female

Lewy Body Dementia
    Male > Female (1.7:1)

Lingual, Facial, and Oromandibular Spasm
    Female > Male

Lumbar Puncture Headache
    Female > Male (2:1)

Lymphoma, Primary Central Nervous System
    Male > Female (slightly)

Madelung's Disease
    Male > Female
    Primarily occurs in males of Mediterranean origin.

Malignant Astrocytoma
    Male > Female (3:2)

Malignant Hyperthermia
   Male > Female

Marchiafava-Bignami Disease (Primary Degeneration of the Corpus Callosum)
   Male > Female
   Occurs in heavy alcohol drinkers.

McCune-Albright Syndrome
   Female > Male

Medulloblastoma
   Male > Female (3:1–2)
   Females have a better survival outcome.

Meningioma
   Female > Male (3:2)
      Adults: more in males in the sixth decade and females in the 7th decade.
   Male = Female
      Childhood

Meningioma (Intracranial)
   Female > Male (1.3:1)
   Often grow during pregnancy due to presence of estrogen and progesterone receptors.

Meningioma (Intraspinal)
   Female > Male

Meningioma of the Sphenoid Ridge
   Female > Male (3:1)

Meningococcal Meningitis
   Male > Female

Menke's Syndrome
   Male > Female

Mental Retardation
   Male > Female (3:1)

Micturition Syncope
   Male > Female

Migraine Headache
   Female > Male (3:1)

After menarche to mid-adult life.
Females also have more frequent attacks.
Peak prevalence age is 45–49 years in females and 40–44 years in males.
- Female > Male (2:1)
    - Postmenopausal
- Male > Female
    - Childhood

Patients with migraines are more likely to have strokes. About 4.6% of males with migraines reported strokes vs. 2.7% of females with migraines.

Males are more likely to have migraine without aura and females are more likely to have migraine with aura.

Females are 2.5 times as likely to have aura without headache than are males.

Females report more pain intensity, greater disability, and more associated symptoms with migraine than men. The duration is longer for females and the median attack rate is higher in females.

Monoclonal Gammopathy of Unknown Significance with Neuropathy
Male > Female

Mononeuritis
Female > Male (2.7:1)

Morton Neuroma
Female > Male (5:1)

Motor Neuropathy with Multifocal Conduction Block
Male > Female (slightly)

Multiple Myeloma with Neuropathy
Male > Female

Multiple Sclerosis
Female > Male (1.7–3:1)

Onset of symptoms appears earlier in females but men tend to exhibit a more progressive and severe disease course. Men usually require assisted walking devices sooner than females. Males also have an increased risk of cerebellar involvement. MS-associated HLA-DR2, DQ6 haplotype is more common in females.

The 10 year mortality rate is higher in males. In affected women, the number of relapses tends to decrease in the third trimester of pregnancy.
The relapsing form of MS occurs predominantly in females.
Women with MS produce more interleukin-5 and interferon-gamma than men with MS.
Sensory or visual dominant pattern is more common in young females.
Males more likely to develop the primary progressive variety and older males have poor prognosis.

Mumps Meningitis
    Male > Female (3:1)

Muscular Dystrophy
    Male > Female
        Duchenne's
        Becker's
        Emery-Dreifuss

Myasthenia Gravis
    Female > Male (3:2)
        Adults: Incidence peaks in the 3rd decade in women and 5th and 6th decades in men. Males seem to have higher rate of thymomas (2.2:1).
    Male ≥ Female
        Elderly
    Female > Male (3:2)
        Children
    Female > Male (5:1)
        Children with myasthenia plus an associated disease.
        If associated with thymoma, then males predominate.

Myotubular Myopathy, X-linked
    Male > Female

Myxedema Coma
    Female > Male
    Primarily occurs in the elderly.

Narcolepsy-Cataplexy Syndrome
    Male > Female

Neonatal Meningitis
   Male > Female (3:1)

Neural Tube Defects
   Female > Male

Neuroblastoma
   Male > Female (0.9–1.4:1)
   Male predominance occurs mainly in children < 5 years of age.

Neurodevelopmental Disorders
   Male > Female

Neurofibromatosis 1
   Females are at higher risk of cancer than males.

Neurolemmoma
   Female > Male

Neuroleptic Malignant Syndrome
   Male > Female (2:1)

Neuropathic Cachexia of Diabetes Mellitus
   Male > Female

Neuropathic Postural Tachycardia Syndrome
   Female > Male
   Usually in young women.

Nonepileptic Seizure
   Female > Male (3.5:1)

Norrie Disease
   Male > Female

Obstructive Sleep Apnea
   Male > Female (2:1)
   Usually obese middle aged males (4%) and females (2%).
   The mean total apnea-hypopnea index (AHI) for total sleep time is higher in men (31 vs. 20 events/hr). Women have a lower AHI NREM (non-rapid eye movement) than men but a similar REM AHI. Obstructive sleep apnea (OSA) is less severe in women because of milder OSA during NREM sleep. Women have a greater clustering of respiratory events during REM sleep. REM OSA is more common in women but supine OSA more common in men.

Occipital Neuralgia
Female > Male

Occult Spinal Dysraphism
Female > Male (2:1)

Oligodendroglioma
Male > Female (2:1)

Orofaciodigital Syndrome
Females only

Osteoarthritis of Cervical Spine
Male > Female

Pain
Women report more pain overall, more severe and chronic pain, in more body regions than men.
Women with osteoarthritis have 40% more pain and severe pain than men but women are more likely to vent their emotions, seek emotional support, and view pain as a warning to slow down. Men are more likely to report negative moods the day after a pain-filled day. Kappa opiod analgesics produce greater and longer-lasting analgesic effects in women than in men.

Paget's Disease
Male > Female (slightly)

Paratrigeminal Syndrome
Male > Female

Parkinson's Disease
Male > Female (1.4:1)
Depressed men, but not women with PD show impairments in both social and physical function.

Pelizaeus-Merzbacher Disease
Male > Female

Pernicious Anemia
Female > Male (1.5:1)

Pheochromocytoma
Female > Male (slightly)

Pinealoma
    Male > Female

Pituitary Adenoma
    Female = Male
    But more clinically evident in females.

Pituitary Apoplexy
    Male > Female (2:1)

Plagiocephaly
    Male > Female

Pneumococcal Meningitis
    Male > Female

Post-Concussive Syndrome
    Male > Female

Postdural Puncture Headache
    Female > Male

Postherpetic Neuralgia
    Male > Female

Posttraumatic Headache
    Male > Female

Primary Amyloid Neuropathy
    Male > Female

Primary Cerebral Lymphoma
    Male > Female

Primary CNS Lymphoma
    Male > Female (slightly)

Progressive Muscular Atrophy
    Male > Female (3.6:1)

Progressive Supranuclear Palsy
    Male > Female (slightly)

Prolactinoma
    Female > Male

Males are relatively insensitive to the affects of prolactin and often will not be diagnosed until the tumor is large and headache or visual symptoms occur.

Males rarely have galactorrha in contrast to females. Males often have impotence, decreased libido and hypogonadism. Females often have menstrual dysfunction, hypoestrogenism, infertility and galactorrhea. The prolactin level and MIB-1 labeling index are lower in young females preoperatively than in males or elderly females.

Males and postmenopausal females usually have macroadenomas at presentation while young females have microadenomas.

Pseudotumor Cerebri
Female > Male (2–4:1)
Primarily overweight adolescents.
Males with psuedotumor cerebri are less likely to be obese than females.
Black men tend to be at greater risk of vision loss.

Rasmussen Encephalitis
Female > Male

Reading Disability
Male > Female (2–5:1)

Recurrent Laryngeal Nerve Paralysis
Male > Female

Relapsing Neuromyelitis Optica
Female > Male (3.8:1)

REM Sleep Behavioral Disorder
Male > Female

Restless Leg Syndrome
Female > Male (slightly)

Rett Syndrome
Females only
X-linked disorder. Believed to be lethal to the hemizygous male in-utero.

Reye's Syndrome
Female > Male (5.2:4.8)

Scaphocephaly
    Female > Male (slightly)

Schwannoma
    Female > Male

Segawa Syndrome (Hereditary Dystonia-Parkinsonism)
    Female > Male (3:2)

Seizure, Absence
    Female > Male (2:1)

Seizure, Febrile
    Male > Female (slightly)

Seizure Disorder, Generalized Tonic-Clonic
    Male > Female (slightly)

Seizure Disorder, Partial
    Male > Female (slightly)

Shy-Drager Syndrome
    Male > Female
    Often in males, the first symptoms are loss of libido and impotence.

Sjaastad's Syndrome
    Female > Male

Sleep Apnea Syndrome
    Male > Female

Spastic Paraplegia, X-linked Type 1
    Male > Female

Spina Bifida
    In birth cohorts of males with spina bifida who had been exposed to prenatal famine, the risk of death was 2.5 times more than in similarly affected female offspring.

Spinal Cord Injury
    Male > Female

Spinal Cord Stroke — AV Fistula
    Male > Female

Spinal Meningioma
>   Female > Male
>   Overall, except higher rate noted in black males.

Spontaneous Dissection of Carotid and Vertebral Arteries
>   Female = Male
>   But occurs on average 5 years earlier in females.

Stiff-Person Syndrome
>   Female > Male
>   Frequently associated with autoimmune disease.

Stroke
>   Male > Female (1–2.4:1)
>   Equalizes after menopause and may be higher in females after age 80 years.
>   Females are more likely to die after stroke at all ages.
>   Females tend to have strokes at a later age than men.
>   Motor, cognitive and functional outcome after stroke may be worse in females.
>   Increased risk of stroke (9 times for ischemic and 28 times for hemorrhagic stroke) during the first 6 weeks after childbirth compared to women of the same age that had not given birth.
>   Females are more likely to have intracranial occlusive disease, especially of the middle cerebral and the intracranial vertebral and posterior cerebral arteries. Males are 2 times as likely to have extracranial occlusive disease, particularly stenoses of the internal carotid artery. Males are more likely (2/3 are male) to have severe internal carotid artery disease.
>   In the Framingham study, the mean age of stroke was 65.4 years in men and 66.1 years in women.
>   Smoking plus oral contraceptives increase the risk of stroke 22 times compared to nonsmoking females using other methods of birth control.
>   A low serum cholesterol (< 10th percentile) is associated with increased intracerebral bleed in elderly men but not young men or women.
>   Diabetes is the most important risk factor for stroke in women, raising a middle aged female's risk to that of age-matched males.
>   Women with diabetes and peripheral vascular disease have a 5 times increased stroke risk and 10 times increased risk for coro-

nary artery disease, but in men only the risk of myocardial infarction (MI) appears to rise.

Atrial fibrillation is associated with a 2 fold stroke risk in men but a 5 fold risk in women.

Aspirin decreases stroke risk by 25% in men and 20% in women. Warfarin appears to have same efficacy in men and women but females have a greater therapeutic response to any given dose.

The risk of stroke is higher in both sexes with migraine headaches (men: 6.8% vs. 4.5%) (women: 3.7% vs. 2.6%) compared to persons without migraine. Male migraineurs have a higher risk of stroke earlier in life than females.

Females are more likely to recover language ability after suffering a left hemispheric stroke.

Women are more likely to suffer depression after stroke than men. Some studies have found a worsened outcome in females with stoke plus a higher total mortality. This may be due to a delay in diagnosis or evaluation of female patients.

Women are more likely to have hemorrhagic strokes (both intracerebral hemorrhage or subarachnoid hemorrhage).

In acute stroke presentation, men are often found to have more traditional stroke symptoms, imbalance and hemiparesis whereas women are found to have more nontraditional stroke symptoms, pain, and change in level of consciousness-disorientation.

For stroke prevention, females undergo fewer angiograms and carotid endarterectomies compared to males.

Stuttering
    Male > Female (3:1)
    And ratio difference increases with age.

Subacute Necrotizing Encephalomyelopathy
    Male > Female

Subarachnoid Hemorrhage
    Female > Male (3:2)
        Overall
        Causes 6–25% of maternal deaths.
    Male > Female
        In persons < 40 years of age.
    Female > Male (3:2)
        In persons > 40 years of age.

Subclavian Steal Syndrome
    Male > Female (2:1)

Subdural Empyema
    Male > Female
    Cases of sinus origin predominate in adolescent and young adult men.

Subdural Hematoma
    Male > Female

Sudden Infant Death Syndrome
    Male > Female (3:2)
    52–60% of cases are males.

Sydenham's Chorea
    Female > Male
    In adolescence, the population is almost exclusively female.

Tabes Dorsalis
    Male > Female

Temporal Arteritis
    Female > Male (2:1)

Tension Headache
    Female > Male (9:7)
            Prevalence: 63%/yr male, 86%/yr in female.
    Episodic Tension Type Headache
        Female > Male (1.16:1)
    Chronic Tension Type Headache
        Female > Male (2.2:1)

Thoracic Outlet Syndrome
    Female > Male (3:1)
        Neurologic Type
    Male > Female
        Venous Type
    Female = Male
        Arterial Type

Thyrotoxicoses with Periodic Paralysis
    Male > Female (20–70:1)

Tic Douloureux
    Female > Male

Torticollis
    Female > Male

Tourette Syndrome
    Male > Female
    1 to 8 cases per 1000 boys
    0.1 to 4 cases per 1000 girls

Transformed Migraine Headache
    Female > Male

Transient Ischemic Attack
    Male > Female (3:1)

Traumatic Head Injury
    Male > Female (2–4:1)
        After age 5 years
    Male = Female
        Up to age 5 years
    Females have improved outcomes compared to males as determined by their ability to return to preinjury work levels.

Trigeminal Neuralgia
    Female > Male (2–3:1)
    Occurs on the right side of the face more often than the left.

Trisomy 13 Syndrome (Patau's Syndrome)
    Female > Male

Trisomy 18 Syndrome (Edwards Syndrome)
    Female > Male

Tuberous Sclerosis
    Male = Female
    But autism is more common in males.

Tussive and Valsalva Syncope
    Male > Female
    Usually is seen in overweight smokers.

Vasculitides
- Polyarteritis Nodosa   1:2.5   F/M
- Churg-Strauss   1:1.4   F/M
- Wegener's   1:1.2   F/M
- Temporal Arteritis   1:2–3   M/F
- Isolated CNS Angiitis   1:2   F/M
- Takayasu's Arteritis   9:1   F/M
- Eales' Disease   Male > Female
- Sneddon's Disease   Female > Male
- Microanginopathy of brain, retina, eye   Female > Male

Venous Angioma with Arterial-Venous Fistula of the Spinal Cord
  Male > Female

Wegener's Granulomatosis
  Male > Female (1.2–2:1)

Whiplash
  Female > Male (2:1)
  Females have persistent neck pain more than men (7:3).
  Possibly due to females having a narrower neck with less muscle mass to support a head of roughly the same volume compared with men.

Cardiology

Anatomy and Physiology

Left Ventricle (LV) mass in males averages 155 ± 18 grams and 110 ± 16 grams in females. The LV end diastolic volume (EDV) in males is 118 ± 27 ml and 96 ± 21 ml in females. The LV end systolic volume (ESV) in males is 40 ± 13 ml and 29 ± 9 ml in females. The Right Ventricle (RV) mass is 52 ± 10 grams in men and 39 ± 5 grams in females. The RV EDV is 131 ± 28 ml in men and 100 ± 23 ml in women. The RV ESV is 53 ± 17 ml in men and 33 ± 15 ml in women. The normal size of the infrarenal aorta is 21.4 mm in men and 18.7 mm in women. Females usually have smaller coronary arteries than men with the same body surface area. The epicardial arterial diameter is about 9% larger in men. Women's heart size is generally smaller than men's. The heart and great vessels weigh 270–360 (average 300) grams in males and 200–280 (average 250) grams in females. Males have greater aortic root dimensions than females. The loss of elasticity and distensibility of the aorta occurs with age, but occurs earlier and is more progressive in males.

Men tend to have higher mean systolic and diastolic blood pressure (BP) than women by 6–7 mm Hg and 3–5 mm Hg respectively. Women have lower mean arterial blood pressure than men before middle age and higher mean arterial blood pressure than men afterwards. While systolic BP is lower in younger women and higher in older women than similarly aged men, the diastolic BP is lower in women throughout adult life. Compared to males with the same level of arterial pressure, females have smaller LV dimensions, higher cardiac output, and lower peripheral resistance, but these changes disappear after menopause. The ankle systolic pressure (ASP) and brachial systolic pressure (BSP) ratio decreases with age in both sexes but in males the decrease in ratio is due to a decrease in ASP whereas BSP does not increase significantly with age. However in females, only BSP correlates with age. Resting supine systolic and diastolic blood pressure is higher in men. Females have decreased small vessel compliance than men despite lower systolic blood pressure. Blood pressure is higher during the follicular phase than the luteal phase in both normotensive and hypertensive women. Aldosterone levels are higher in women than men during the luteal phase but not during the preovulatory phase of menses. Males have higher mean renin levels than women.

Baroreflex sensitivity (BRS): Decreases with age in men whereas in females it plateaus during the 5th decade of life, thus BRS is higher in females after age 60 years old.

Heart rate (normal resting):
    Males: 46–93 beats per minute
    Females: 51–95 beats per minute
    Heart rate is faster in all ages of females compared to males.

The average resting heart rate for women while asleep is 66 beats per minute (bpm) and 90 bpm while awake. For males, the average heart rate while asleep is 56 bpm and 80 bpm while awake. The faster basal heart rate in women is mainly due to differences in exercise capacity and not to intrinsic properties of the sinus node. The sinus node recovery time is longer in males. Males are more likely to display carotid sinus hypersensitivity.

With exercise, males increase left ventricular ejection fraction while females increase left ventricle volume to increase the cardiac output. Evaluation of heart rate before and after exercise in healthy volunteers shows men to have a longer average sinus cycle length than women after autonomic influences are blocked. Females may have a greater parasympathetic modulation of heart rate, and it appears to be modulated by hormones. Healthy females in their 20's have higher rates of premature ventricular beats (54% vs. 50%) and atrial premature beats (64% vs. 56%) than males of the same age. Boys appear to have a higher cardiac reactivity to a stressful stimulus than girls.

Basal vasopressin secretion is higher in men than women, and in blacks than whites. Males have lower mean tissue plasminogen activator (t-PA) activity but higher plasminogen activator inhibitor (PAI) levels than females. Males have higher urokinase plaminogen activator levels. Males have higher t-PA and PAI antigen levels than females. The density of peripheral vascular adrenergic receptors is lower in women than men.

Creatine Kinase Levels:
    Male: 1.00–6.67 ukat/liter
    Female: 0.67–2.50 ukat/liter

Gender Differences in Hemodynamic Response to Exercise

Criteria	Men	Women
Left Ventricular Ejection Fraction	++ (most) + (some)	0 (many)
Left Ventricular End-Systolic Vol.	- (most) - (some)	0 (most)
Left Ventricular End-Diastolic Vol.	0 (most) - (some)	+ (most) 0 (some)
Systolic Blood Pressure	++++	+++

Compared to men, women have a smaller rest end-diastolic index (87 versus 97 ml/m^2) and a greater increase in end-diastolic volume with exercise. Men tend to have a lower rest ejection fraction than women (0.63 versus 0.66) and a greater increase in ejection fraction with exercise (0.08 versus 0.02) The VO$_2$ max is 6.2% higher in boys than girls and the maximal stroke volume is 5.2% greater in boys. At puberty the gender gap in VO$_2$ max widens and is 25-30% higher in men at age 18 years than in women of that age. Females have a smaller heart size, a diminished rise in exercise ejection fraction and a lower maximal cardiac output than men. Left ventricular mass is greater in men than in women as a result of larger chamber size in men and patterns of hypertrophy. Females have greater systolic chamber function but lower diastolic compliance of the LV. With exercise, LV stroke volume change in females occurs by increasing the LVEDV with little change in the LV ejection fraction between rest and maximum exercise, but in males the LV ejection fraction increases with little change in the LVEDV. The maximal arterial-venous oxygen difference is about 20% greater in adult men.

Atrial natriuetic peptide (ANP) levels are two times higher in young women than young men. However no difference in ANP is noted in menopausal women and age-matched men. Young females have higher levels of nuclear-localized phospho-Akt (a protein kinase) in myocardial cells compared to young men or postmenopausal women. Estrogen receptors are higher in varicose segments than nonvaricose segments of the same vein, especially in females. Progesterone receptor levels are denser in nonvaricose segments of females than in those of males.

Pulse pressure is higher in males until age 55 years, after which it becomes higher in females of similar age. Women develop a higher degree of arterial pulsatility with aging, despite lower mean blood pressure and similar arterial distensibility. Baroreceptor reflex sensitivity is lower and heart rate variability of parasympathetic markers is higher in women, except BRS tends to be higher in women > 60 years old.

During cold exposure where cardiac output increases in both sexes, men achieve an increase in cardiac output by slower heart rates and increased stroke volume and VO_2, but these changes are not seen in women. Women do not show a heart rate-stroke volume shift in either resting or exercising states in cold environments. During supine exercise, the ejection fraction increases more in males and the end-diastolic volume index is more increased in females. Men have a greater percentage of decline in end-systolic volume with exercise.

Women are more sensitive than men to fluctuations in coronary vasomotor tone. Cardiac repolarization is shorter and faster in men. Testosterone appears to play a role in modulating cardiac repolarization. Men appear to be more subject to oxidative stresses than women. Young women have lower lipid peroxidation levels than young men. Females have higher levels of vascular endothelial growth factor at all ages than males. Norepinephrine causes less forearm vasoconstriction in women than men. Stimulation of beta-2 adrenergic receptors causes more forearm vasodilation in women.

EKGs done on 1450 young healthy adults found that females tend to have a faster heart rate, shortened conduction times (PQ, Q, ventricular activation time and QRS) and prolonged repolarization time (QTc), decreased P, Q, and T amplitudes as well as indices of right, septal and left ventricular hypertrophy. The ST elevation in precordial leads was lower in women than men. Sinus bradycardia was more common in men, but sinus tachycardia was more common in females. AV block grade 1 was found in 1% of females and 3% of males. Notching of R/S in V1-V2 and incomplete Right bundle branch block were less common in women. Women normally have slightly longer QT intervals than men (420 ± 17 ms vs. 400 ± 20 ms). This difference is not seen in childhood. At puberty, the QT interval decreases in boys but remains the same in girls, suggesting male hormones may be responsible for the difference. Longer QT intervals occur at rest and with exercise in adult women.

Cardioverter-defibrillators appear more effective in women, because of the generally lower defibrillation thresholds in women.

Diseases

Abdominal Aortic Aneurysm
> Male > Female (2.3–5:1)
> Occurs in 2–5% of men > 60 years; 6% of men > 65 years; 11% of men > 75 years of age.
> Occurs in 4% of women > 65 years of age.
> Mortality rate in people with aortic abdominal aneurysm is 4.5 times greater in men. Aneurysm rupture is cause of death in 1.2% of men and 0.6% of women.
> Incidence is increasing; male siblings are at risk (up to 12 fold risk). Incidence increases after age 55 years in males and 70 years in females.
> Women with abdominal aortic aneurysms are older and appear to have a higher risk of rupture (up to 4 times higher), higher rupture-related mortality, and higher mortality after elective repair.

Accessory A-V Pathways
> Male > Female (2:1)
> Spontaneous orthodromic tachycardia is more frequent in females (1.3:1), while atrial and ventricular fibrillation is more common in males.

Acute Pericarditis
> Male > Female

Alcoholic Cardiomyopathy
> Male > Female
> Males are usually heavy consumers for more than 10 years.
> Female alcoholics who develop cardiomyopathy appear to have a lower cumulative lifetime dose of alcohol than male alcoholics with cardiomyopathy.
> Subclinical LV dysfunction is common in male but rare in female alcoholics.

Angina Pectoris
> Male > Female

This is the presenting symptom of coronary artery disease in 38% of men and 61% of women.

Women are more likely to present with angina as their initial manifestation of coronary artery disease (CAD).

50% of females referred for angiography do not have significant stenosis, compared to only 17% of males.

Microvascular spasms are more common in females.

Males are two times more likely to have MI within five years of angina onset.

CAD death rate is 40–50% higher in men at 2 and 10 years after onset of angina compared to women.

In females with typical exertional angina symptoms, the incidence of coronary artery disease is less than in men with typical symptoms, 70% vs. 90%.

The Asn291Ser substitution in lipoprotein lipase is associated with increased plasma triglyceride levels and a 2 times increase in risk of ischemic heart disease in women but not men.

Females are more likely to experience anginal pain at rest, during sleep, or with mental stress.

Females have more vasospastic angina and microvascular angina.

Angiosarcoma of the Heart
Male > Female (2:1)

This is in contrast to most other cardiac sarcomas that have no sex preference.

Annuloaortic Ectasia
Male > Female

Aortic Arch Calcification
Female > Male

Independently related to coronary heart disease risk in both sexes as well as to ischemic stroke risk in women. About 10.6% of men and 15.9% of women over age 65 years have aortic arch calcification.

Aortic Coarctation
Male > Female (2:1)

Aortic Dissection
Male > Female (2–3:1)

Half of dissections in females under age 40 occur in women who are pregnant.
Several cases reported in male cocaine users.

Aortic Regurgitation
A dystrophic etiology is more common in males.

Aortic Valvular Stenosis
Male > Female
    < Age 60 years
Female > Male
    Elderly
Congenital bicuspid valve: Male > Female (4:1)
Congenital unicuspid valve: Male > Female (3:1)
With comparable degrees of AS, men manifest a greater increase in LV wall mass with cavity dilatation, while women show greater increases in wall thickening. Elderly women show more marked concentric hypertrophy, lower levels of wall stress, and higher indexes of systolic function than elderly men with aortic stenosis.
Evaluation for AS typically occurs later in life in elderly females than elderly males resulting in more frequent and higher-risk emergency surgery in females.

Aortoiliac Vascular Disease
Male > Female
    Overall
Male > Female (2:1)
    Young population
Male > Female (10–15:1)
    Elderly population

Arrhythmia
Females may have a lower defibrillation threshold and higher rate of resuscitation from ventricular tachycardia or ventricular fibrillation than males.
Electrophysiologic testing is less sensitive and less specific in females.
Premature ventricular contractions after MI are risk factors for sudden death in men.
Proarrhythmia drug-induced torsades de pointes is more common in females.

Females report subjective sense of palpitations and irregular heart beat more than males.

Females in ages 20–30's have more atrial and ventricular ectopic beats than men of the same age.

Overall, asymptomatic frequent or complex ventricular arrhythmias are more common in males.

Sudden death is more common in males (3:1). The risk of sudden death is delayed 20 years for females.

In patients without previous clinical evidence of CAD, the traditional risk factors for CAD such as age, weight, cholesterol level, LVH, smoking are not predictive for sudden death in females but they are in males.

Many studies show a correlation between longer QT interval and mortality in males post-MI.

Accessory pathways are more common in males.

Arrhythmia, Ventricular Tachycardia
   Male > Female (5:2)
   Ventricular arrhythmias in elderly occur in 25% of men and 15% of women.

Arrhythmogenic Right Ventricular Cardiomyopathy
   Male > Female

Arterial Disease of the Lower Extremities
   Male > Female

Arterial Embolus and Thrombosis
   Male > Female

Arteriosclerotic Heart Disease
   Male > Female
   Predominant age for clinical manifestations: Male 50–60 years; Females 60–70 years.
   In diabetic males, there is a 2–3 times increased risk of cardiovascular disease, but a 3–4 times increased risk in female diabetics. Also diabetic females have a twofold higher risk of mortality from myocardial infarction and congestive heart failure.
   Obesity results in increased coronary heart disease risk in females. Females have slightly higher mortality and morbidity from cardiovascular disease.

Angina from microvascular disease and vasospasm, and chest pain precipitated by panic attacks and anxiety are more common in females.

Younger women with infarcts are more likely to have higher complication and death rates than young men with infarcts.

Women are also more likely to have non-Q wave infarcts.

In men, the three main presentations of coronary heart disease—angina, sudden death, myocardial infarction—are equally distributed while in women angina is the most common manifestation.

Females are twice as likely to present with angina as men and less likely to present with infarction or sudden death.

Women are more likely to complain of dyspnea, fatigue, back, shoulder and arm pain. Women are less likely than men to think that their pain is cardiac in origin.

Acutely, following an infarction, women are more likely to have heart failure and cardiogenic shock.

Males with infarcts are more likely to have ST segment elevation on the EKG.

Calcium deposits in coronary arteries are associated with a 50% higher risk of blood-clot related stroke in women, but elevated stroke risk not seen in men.

Among people with MI, men more often present with ventricular tachycardia and women more often present with cardiogenic shock and cardiac arrest.

The use of lipid-lowering agents (certain statins) may be more beneficial in females in overall reduction in sudden death, nonfatal MI and stroke and beneficial effects may be noticed sooner in females after beginning therapy.

Lifetime Cumulative Risk of Developing Coronary Heart Disease

Age	Male	Female
40	49%	32%
50	50%	31%
60	43%	29%
70	35%	24%

Pretest Likelihood (%) of Coronary Artery Disease

Age	Asymptomatic		Nonanginal		Atypical Angina		Typical Angina	
	M	F	M	F	M	F	M	F
35–44	3.7	0.7	10.5	2.7	42.8	15.5	80.9	45.4
45–54	7.7	2.1	20.6	6.9	60.1	31.7	90.7	67.7
55–64	11.1	5.4	28.2	12.7	69	46.5	93.9	83.9
65–74	11.3	11.5	28.2	17.1	70	54.1	94.3	94.7

Typical = substernal chest pain, precipitated by exertion, relieved within 10 minutes of rest or nitroglycerin
Atypical = positive to two of the three symptoms
Nonangina = positive to one of three
Asymptomatic = no complaints of discomfort in the chest

Atheroembolism
- Male > Female

Atherosclerosis
- Male > Female
- Cereal fiber appears to have a stronger apparent effect in females in protecting against coronary heart disease.
- Age > 45 years confers increased risk in men compared to > 55 years in women.
- The risk for coronary heart disease increases in women with HDL values < 45 mg/dl and < 35 mg/dl in men. VLDL triglyceride levels are a greater independent risk factor in females. LDL tends to plateau in men after age 50 years but continues to rise after menopause in females.

Atherosclerotic Occlusive Disease
- Male > Female (2:1)
- Signs and symptoms of coronary artery disease occur about 10 years earlier in men.
- Complications after percutaneous transluminal coronary angioplasty are more common in females (29% vs. 20%). Females are more likely to have angina after a PTCA and higher mortality rate than men but more likely to report their angina as less severe. However after coronary artery bypass surgery, females may have better long term survival.
- The 1998 age-adjusted death rate in men compared to women ≥ 35 years of age from coronary heart disease was 222.4 vs. 135.8 per 100,000 and 99.7 vs. 58.8 per 100,000 for acute myocardial infarction.
- However in patients younger than age 50 years, females are more likely to die after an MI.
- Smoking seems to cause more carotid and femoral artery intima-media thickening in males than females.

Atrial Fibrillation
> Male > Female
> Annual incidence per 1000 person-years in adults age 55–64 years is 3.1 cases in males and 1.9 cases in females. Over age 65 years, the frequency is 6.2% of males and 4.8% of females.
> Mortality associated with atrial fibrillation is greater in women (Odds Ratio 1.9 vs. 1.5).
> More common in males after cardiac surgery.
> If AF developed after an MI, long-term follow-up shows that males had a 50% increased risk of death and females had a 90% increased risk.
> In females with nonvalvular AF, warfarin reduced stroke risk by 84% compared to 60% in males. Females treated with aspirin had stroke risk reduction of 23% versus 44% in males.
> Women have a higher heart rate at the onset of AF compared to men (123/min vs 115 /min). Women also have a higher heart rate during an episode of AF and the duration of AF tends to be longer in females (90 vs 50 minutes). Women are also somewhat more difficult to maintain in sinus rhythm after cardioversion.
> More women with AF have underlying valvular disease, whereas more men have underlying coronary artery disease.
> MI increases the risk of AF in males by 40%.
> Women are more likely to develop drug-induced arrhythmias when medically treated for AF.
> The frequency of AF is increasing in males but not females. This may be due to improved survival after MI.
> Women that smoke are 1.4 times more likely to develop AF than male smokers.
> Embolic events occur in 14% of females and 6% of males with nonrheumatic AF.
> Women have a higher incidence of major bleeds when treated with warfarin for AF.

Atrial Myxoma
> Female > Male (7:3)

Atrial Reentrant Tachycardia
> Female > Male

Atrial Septal Defect
> Female > Male (2:1)

Atrioventricular Nodal Reentrant Tachycardia
Female > Male (2:1)

Bicuspid Aortic Valve
Male > Female (4:1)
Adults

Cardiac Amyloidosis
Male > Female

Cardiac Arrest
Male > Female (4–5:1)
45% of female compared to 80% of male survivors of out of hospital cardiac arrest had coronary artery disease.
A LV ejection fraction of < 40% is a predictor of cardiac mortality in men but not women.

Cardiac Transplant
Male > Female (4:1)
CAD is etiology of 30% of females undergoing transplant compared to 50% of males.
Females possibly have lower survival post-transplant.
Female gender is a risk factor for rejection of cardiac transplant.
Patients with severe LV dysfunction on a nonischemic basis are more likely male.

Cardiomyopathy
Cardiomyopathy seems to be tolerated better in females than males.
Hyperdynamic hypertrophic cordiomyopathy of the elderly usually occurs in females.
Women with hypertrophic cardiomyopathy have a smaller left ventricular cavity size than men which predisposes to LV outflow obstruction.

Gender Associated Cardiomyopathy
1) Postpartum: Females only
2) Duchenne's Muscular Dystrophy: Male > Female
3) Becker's Muscular Dystrophy: Male > Female

Carney's Syndrome
Female > Male (1.8:1)

Carotid Sinus Syndrome
   Male > Female (2:1)

Chronic Heart Failure
   Male > Female (3.7:2.4)
   Risk of CHF is higher in females after MI.
   The 5 year survival is greater in females with CHF than males with CHF (38% vs 25%).
   Hypertension (HTN) and diabetes (DM) are greater risk factors for CHF in men.
   Females develop CHF more frequently following an MI.
   Risk of developing CHF in females with diabetes is higher than in males with diabetes.
   Underlying cause of CHF is more frequently CAD in men versus DM, HTN and atrial fibrillation in females.

Chronic Venous Insufficiency
   Female > Male

Claudication
   Male > Female (4:1)
   Common in Males > 55 years; Females > 60 years

Coarctation of the Aorta
   Male > Female (1.7–3:1)
      Adult

Complete Atrioventricular Canal
   Female > Male

Complicating Myocardial Infarction
   Female > Male

Congenital Aneurysm of an Aortic Sinus of Valsalva
   Male > Female (3:1)

Congenital Heart Disease
   Male > Female (overall)
      Valvular Aortic Stenosis   Male > Female (4:1)
      Pulmonary and Tricuspid Atresia   Male > Female
      Discrete Subaortic Stenosis   Male > Female (2:1)
      Patent Ductus Arteriosus   Female > Male (2–3:1)
      Congenital Bicuspid Aortic Valve Male > Female (4:1)

Congenital Unicuspid Aortic Valve	Male > Female (3:1)
Ebstein's Anomaly of the Tricuspid	Female > Male
Atrial Septal Defect	Female > Male (2:1)
Coarctation of Aorta	Male > Female
Hypoplasia of Left Heart	Male > Female (2:1)
Congenital Pericardial Defect	Male > Female
Tetraology of Fallot	Male > Female
Transposition of the Great Vessels	Male > Female (2:1)

In females with congenital heart disease, age of menarche is slightly delayed (~ 1 year) compared to controls.

Preexisting cardiac failure often becomes more severe during pregnancy in females with congenital heart disease.

Females with Eisenmenger syndrome have increased risk of thromboembolism during pregnancy.

With congenital heart disease, especially cyanotic type, boys appear to be retarded more in growth than girls, especially in the second decade of life.

Congenital Heart Disease in Adults

Frequency of Occurrence in Adults		% Adult Female
1st	Ventricular Septal Defect	54%
2nd	Pulmonic Stenosis	50%
3rd	Atrial Septal Defect	70%
4th	Aortic Stenosis	20%
5th	Tetralogy of Fallot	49%
6th	Coarctation of Aorta	36%
7th	AV Septal Defect	56%
8th	Patent Ductus Arteriosus	82%
9th	Tricuspid/Pulmonic Atresia	54%
10th	Complete Transposition	30%

Congenital Long QT Syndrome

Female > Male (3:2)

Female sex is an independent risk factor for syncope and sudden death.

In men, the risk for first cardiac event is usually higher in childhood and decreases after puberty.

Females with the condition are at significant risk for cardiac events during the postpartum period. This increased risk may be due to an increase in sympathetic activity or to higher levels of estrogen and progesterone that may influence (directly or indirectly) the number and function of mutant ion channel proteins.

Congenital Pericardial Defects
    Male > Female
    Usually occurs on the left side.
    60% of cases occur in females.

Congestive Heart Failure
    Male > Female (4:3)
        Overall
    Male > Female
        Ages 40–75 years
    Male = Female
        Ages older than 75 years
Over the last 50 years, the incidence of CHF has decreased in women but not men, but the survival has increased in both sexes.
Congestive heart failure tends to occur earlier in men.
Death rate from CHF for persons > 65 years is greater for males than females.
Women with advanced CHF survive twice as long as men.
If the cause of the heart failure is non-ischaemic, women survive 3 times longer but if the etiology is ischaemic, the advantage is only half as large.
Hypertension induced heart failure is more common in females (34% vs. 21%).
Females develop CHF at higher LV ejection fraction than males.
Females with CHF live longer than males with CHF.
The risk of developing thrombotic events may be greater in females with CHF.
Women have a greater functional incapacity for the same degree of left ventricle dysfunction.
Females have a higher prevalence of diastolic dysfunction.
Diabetes appears to promote heart failure to a larger extent in females.
Males with CHF are more likely than females to have coronary artery disease.
Females with CHF more likely to have valvular disease and hypertensive heart disease.
Females develop CHF at an older age than males.

CHF after myocardial infarction is more common in females.
Females with diabetes mellitus have more left ventricular hypertrophy than males with diabetes mellitus.
Females with hypertension have greater degree of LVH than men with HTN.
Females with nonischemic CHF have an attenuated sympathetic activation and parasympathetic withdrawal compared to men.

Coronary Artery Bypass Grafting
Mortality is 1.4–4.4 times higher in females. In females, mortality is 3.9% vs. 2.3% in men. In addition, females are less likely to receive internal mammary artery graft or complete revascularization and are more likely to experience complications of heart failure, perioperative infarction, and hemorrhage.
Females undergoing CABG are more likely to have preserved ventricular function and are less likely to have multivessel disease.
Females are more likely to have urgent or emergency CABG.
Females are less likely to be free of angina post-CABG and experience greater disability and are less likely to return to work.
Long term survival after CABG: Women die of myocardial infarction and CHF, while men die of sudden death or cancer.
Females are more likely to have angina after CABG than males 40–45% vs. 30–35%, but females report angina is more manageable than males.

Coronary Artery Disease
Male > Female
Females acquire disease 6–10 years later than men.
Females have myocardial infarctions at an older age than men (about 20 years later).
Angina—Men (25%) develop MI with symptoms compared to 14% of women.
Women with coronary artery disease are more likely to present with angina.
Mortality rate after MI is worse in females than males. The 1 year mortality rate after 1st MI is 45% in females vs 10% in males.
In hospital mortality rate for MI is higher in females.
Reinfarction rate in females > males within days after MI.
Reinfarction rate within 1 year is 40% in females versus 13% in males.

Cardiology

Female with typical angina have CAD only 50% of the time compared to 83% of men with typical angina.

Female diabetics have an increased cardiovascular disease risk two times that of male diabetics.

There is a higher incidence of obesity, hypertension and dyslipidemia in female diabetics.

Females with CAD seem to have more DM, hypertension, and increased cholesterol compared to males with CAD.

Retinal arteriolar narrowing is a risk factor for CAD in women but not men, thus supporting a more prominent microvascular role in development of CAD in women than men.

Coronary Artery Disease in Women

Dietary intervention for dyslipidemia may be less effective in women.

Diabetes increases mortality of myocardial infarct more in women.

Obesity and body fat distribution appear to be more important risk factors for CAD in women.

The reported beneficial effects of exercise on CAD risk profile are less marked in females compared with males, with lesser increases in HDL and less weight loss resulting from similar exercise training.

Females are more likely to present with angina and are less likely to present with MI (compared to males) as the first or subsequent manifestation of CAD.

Females are on average 5–10 years older at the time of presentation.

Females with chronic angina are older and more likely to have hypertension, diabetes and CHF, but are less likely to have had a prior MI or revascularization than males.

The resting EKG reveals a higher prevalence of repolarization (ST-T wave) abnormalities in females with suspected coronary disease than in men with suspected CAD (32% vs. 23%).

Treadmill exercise testing has higher false positive rates in females (38–67%) than in males (7–44%).

Females are more likely than males to experience vascular and renal complications during diagnostic angiography, possibly due to older age, more diabetes, and smaller body size.

Females have higher mortality after balloon angioplasty.

Surgical mortality of left main coronary vessel disease is 2 times higher in females.

Acute and long term coronary graft patency after bypass appears lower in females.

Long term survival after CABG: females die of MI and CHF while males die from sudden death or cancer.

1 in 17 females vs. 1 in 5 males have a coronary event by age 50.

Initial presentation of CAD as myocardial infarction is less common in females but the initial episode of MI in females are more likely fatal and late survival and morbidity worse in females (1 year mortality is 45% in females vs. 10% in males).

Early reinfarction is more common in females, and females have more unrecognized infarctions than males (35% vs. 27%)

Cardiac rupture occurs more often in females with MI.

Females undergoing CABG have higher prevalence of CHF symptoms than men.

The rate of severe CAD in persons undergoing coronary angiography for MI is worse in males than females.

ECG stress test has lower positive predictive value in females. Females have more false positive and nondiagnostic results.

Radionuclide angiocardigraphy also has more false positive results in females.

Radionuclide myocardial perfusion imaging has more false positive and false negative results in females.

Coronary Heart Failure
> Male > Female
>> < 75 years
> Female > Male
>> > 75 years
>
> Males with CHF are more likely to have coronary artery disease.
> Females with CHF are more likely to have valvular disease and hypertensive heart disease.
> Female survival > Male with coronary heart failure.
> Females develop coronary heart failure at an older age than males.
> Coronary heart failure after myocardial infarction is more common in females.
> Increased hematocrit is risk factor for CHF in females.
> Females have greater degree of LVH with hypertension than males.
> With exercise, males increase LV ejection fraction while females increase LV volume to increase cardiac output.

Cor Pulmonale
> Male > Female

Deep Venous Thrombosis
  Female > Male (1.2:1)

Depression in Coronary Heart Disease
  Female > Male
  Risk of depression with coronary heart disease is twice as high in females as that of males.

Digitalis Toxicity
  Female > Male

Dilated Cardiomyopathy
  Male > Female
  60–90% are male.
  The long-term outcome and prognostic factors in these diseases show no sex differences.

Emery-Dreifuss Muscular Dystrophy
  Male > Female
  Associated with cardiac conduction abnormalities.

Endocardial Fibroelastosis
  Male > Female

Endocarditis
  Male > Female (1.6–2.5:1)
  In rheumatic heart disease, endocarditis is more likely to affect mitral valve in women and the aortic valve in men.
  A bicuspid aortic valve is a common site for endocarditis in males.

Fabry Disease
  Male > Female

Familial Pulmonary Hypertension
  Female > Male

Femoral and Popliteal Artery Aneurysm
  Male > Female (20–30:1)
  These constitute 90% of all periperal aneurysms.

Fragile-X Syndrome
Male > Female
Aortic root dilation and mitral valve prolapse seen.

Giant Cell Arteritis
Female > Male (2–3:1)
Females that have murmurs in their arteries or that smoke are more likely to have or develop giant cell arteritis than men with similar traits.

Heart Disease
Black females tend to have accelerated organ changes, especially of the kidney.
Blacks respond poorly to Beta-Blockers.
Females with heart disease are more likely to have DM and hypertension than males.
Hyperinsulinemia has been targeted as a promoter of atherosclerosis in males, but not females.

Heart Disease in the Elderly
In the Framingham Heart Study, males developed coronary artery disease at a younger age (37% in males 65–74 years old versus 22% in females of similar age). Between age 75–84 years, 44% of males and 28% of females had CAD, in the 85–94 year group 48% of males and 43% of females had CAD.
CAD mortality is about two times as great in males.
Hypertension—56% of males and 61% of females by age 65–74 years and 64% of males and 77% of females age > 75 years have high blood pressure (defined as at least one ambulatory BP reading ≥ 140/90)
Smoking—15% of males and 11.5% of females ≥ 65 years smoke.
Cholesterol—22% of males and 41% of females age 65–74 years had total serum cholesterol >240 mg/dl. Whereas 20% of males and 38% of females >75 years had total serum cholesterol >240 mg/dl.
Physical inactivity—38% of males and 51% of females >75 years report no leisure time activity.
Of patients with heart failure < age 65 years, most are male, while 60% of patients with heart failure over age 65 years are females.

Henoch-Schonlein Purpura
> Male > Female (2:1)
> Most common vasculitis seen in children.
> Renal involvement more common in males.

Hepatic Artery Aneurysm
> Male > Female (2:1)

HLA B-27 Associated Spondyloarthropathies
> Male > Female
> Males are more likely to have conduction abnormalities.

Hyperdynamic Hypertrophic Cardiomyopathy of the Elderly
> Female > Male
> Usually in females
> Digitalis toxicity is more common in females.

Hyperlipidemia
> After age 25 years, the cholesterol level rises next 20 years in both sexes, then plateaus, but females have higher cholesterol level at age 45–50 years. The level then exceeds males by 20–25 points for the duration of life.
> HDL is higher in females than males from puberty until menopause. Afterwards, the HDL level then declines along with a rise in total cholesterol levels.
> Triglyceride levels rise more slowly in females than males. The triglyceride level is similar in males and females by age 65–70 years. Low HDL tends to be a more powerful predictor of CAD in females than males.
> Triglyceride levels appear to convey a higher CAD risk in females.

Hypertension
> Male > Female (1.25:1)
>> Until middle age
> Female > Male
>> In elderly
> After age 60 years, the age-associated increase in blood pressure is more pronounced in females and at advanced age, hypertension is more prevalent among females.
> Males seem to have higher mean systolic (by 6–7 mm Hg) and diastolic (by 3–5 mm Hg) pressures until age 60 years than females,

and men have a higher risk of cardiovascular disease at any given pressure.

Systolic BP is lower in females in early adulthood, but the rate of increase is steeper and results in BP levels as high or higher than those in men after age 60.

Women have lower average diastolic BP than men at all ages.

Elderly women and men with hypertension tend to have increased peripheral resistance, low or normal plasma volume, and low plasma renin levels.

In contrast with men, younger females tend to have higher cardiac indexes, heart rates, and left ventricular ejection times but a lower total peripheral resistance, blood volume and blood pressure increase with stress.

Middle-age males with systolic hypertension appear to have higher risk of death when their diastolic blood pressure is normal than when it is mildly elevated. However women tend to have a higher risk of death when both the systolic and diastolic blood pressure are elevated.

Postmenopausal females appear to have higher risk for hypertension than men and more women die of hypertension than men.

Hypertension causes stroke more often in women (59% vs. 39%) and is a stronger risk factor for the development of CHF (hazard ratio 3.2 vs. 2.0) in females.

Women are more likely to have white coat hypertension.

Women are more likely to have salt sensitive hypertension if they have a family history of hypertension.

Women who receive treatment for hypertension may have more side effects than men. Diuretic induced hyponatremia and hypokalemia may be more common in women than in men. ACE inhibitor-associated cough is 2–3 times more common in women than in men.

Sexual dysfunction due to antihypertensive therapy is more common in men than women.

Women with hypertension have lower systolic and diastolic intraarterial blood pressures (IABPs) than men. Women also have a greater nocturnal fall in systolic and diastolic IABPs and they have greater long term systolic and diastolic IABP variability and heart rate variability than men.

Heart rate variability reduction is associated with increased likelihood of hypertension in men but not women.

Male, but not female, offspring of HTN parents have modified diastolic function and autonomic control of heart rate.

Sodium-lithium countertransport is higher in men than women between 20–59 years of age.

Erythrocyte sodium is associated with hypertension in women but not men.

The rate of ouabain-sensitive sodium efflux is higher in males.

Females have greater increase in hypertension risk with increasing baseline diastolic BP and weight gain than do men.

Elderly women are more NaCl sensitive than men.

Weight is a better predictor for hypertension in girls than in boys.

Women are more likely to be aware that they are hypertensive, to be receiving antihypertensive medicine, and to have their blood pressure controlled.

B-adrenergic blockers tend to be less effective in women than men.

Women are more susceptible to ACE-I induced cough, calcium channel blocker induced edema and minoxidil induced hirsutism.

Females have a greater risk of HTN with worsening glucose tolerance.

Females tolerate hypertension better than males, with a longer delay in most cardiovascular complications including development of LVH.

Young premenopausal women are half as likely to express the non-modulating phenotype of essential HTN as men but no gender differences seen in postmenopausal women.

Black females tend to have accelerated organ changes, especially of the kidneys.

Blacks respond poorly to Beta-blockers and better to diuretics and calcium blockers.

For a given increment in systolic BP, the prevalence of LVH is higher in males than females.

Women with essential HTN have higher resting heart rate, cardiac index, and pulse pressure but lower total peripheral resistance than men with the same pressure level.

Normal women have lower left ventricle mass than men. Under age 50, males have more LVH than females; the converse is true among older people.

Compared with men with the same level of arterial pressure, females have smaller LV dimension, higher cardiac output, and lower peripheral resistance, but these differences tend to disappear after menopause.

Women have a lower incidence of CHF than men at the same blood pressure level, possibly because they are hemodynamically younger for any given blood pressure level.

The risk of developing hypertension is greater in obese females than in obese males.

Alcohol intake is an independent predictor of hypertension in males and females, and associated with LV mass in males but not females. End-stage renal disease in hypertension has a higher incidence rate in men.

Hemodynamic Measurements at Peak Exercise in Hypertensive Persons

Measurement	Male	Female
Work Load (Watts)	154 ± 35	87 ± 23
Oxygen Uptake (L/min)	2.09 ± 0.40	1.48 ± 0.40
Cardiac Output (L/min)	16.1 ± 3.8	13.4 ± 3.8
Stroke Volume (ml)	97.6 ± 22.6	77.8 ± 22.6
Heart rate (beats/min)	171 ± 21	167 ± 17
(AV)O_2 (ml/liter)	133 ± 22.3	108 ± 16.0
Hemoglobin (g/dl)	16.5 ± 1.3	14.3 ± 1.3

(The difference in VO_2 was due to smaller stroke volume and lower peak arteriovenous oxygen content difference among the women)

Hypertensive Emergencies
Male > Female

Hypertensive Hypertrophic Cardiomyopathy
Female > Male
Usually in elderly females.

Hypertrophic Cardiomyopathy
Male > Female (slightly)
Females may be more likely to be severely disabled and may present initially at a younger age than males.

Idiopathic Aortitis
Female > Male (2:1)

Idiopathic Dilated Cardiomyopathy
Male > Female
Survival is less in males.
Women often present at a more advanced stage of disease with greater LV dilation.

Infective Endocarditis
- Male > Female (1.6–2.5:1)
- In one study, 1.7 and 1.2 per 100,000 male and female children respectively had infective endocarditis.
- In rheumatic heart disease, in females the mitral valve is more commonly affected. Whereas in males, the aortic valve is more commonly affected than in females.
- Enterococcal infections usually occur in young females or elderly males.
- Men with mitral valve prolapse and systolic murmur are at a higher risk for development of IE than females with mitral valve prolapse.
- IV drug users with IE are more likely male (3:1).

Ischemic Cardiomyopathy
- Male > Female

Isolated Systolic Hypertension
- Female > Male

Kawasaki's Disease
- Male > Female (1.5:1)
- Males are more likely to develop coronary aneurysms.

Klinefelter's Syndrome
- Males only
- Possible conduction abnormalities and increased venous thromboembolic disease.

Left Ventricular Hypertrophy
- More eccentric in men and more concentric in women.
- Weight and obesity are more important in the development of LVH in women than in men.
- Isolated systolic hypertension is more likely to result in the development of LVH in women than in men.
- LVH in women is associated with more cardiovascular risk than in men with similar degrees of LVH (2.1 vs. 1.9).
- In response to an increase in pressure, women develop concentric LVH (increased LV wall thickness and mass) without chamber enlargement whereas males do not generate increased wall thickness but generate more muscle mass through LV dilation.

For comparative degrees of aortic stenosis, women develop concentric LVH and have better contractile parameters than men. Women's dP/dt is better, and cardiac index higher than men's. In contrast men have higher mean pulmonary artery pressure and three times more subnormal ejection performance with aortic stenosis.

Loffler's Disease
    Male > Female

Loffler's Endocarditis Parietalis Fibroplastica
    Male > Female

Long QT Syndrome
    Female > Male

Lymphedema, Praecox and Tarda
    Female > Male (2–9:1)

Marfan's Syndrome
    Male = Female
    But females are more likely to have mitral valve prolapse.
    Males tend to die before females by about 10 years.
    Males have aortic insufficiency and aortic dissection more than females.
    Females have mitral valve prolapse and mitral regurgitation more than males.

Mesenteric Venous Thrombosis
    Male > Female (slightly)

Microvascular Angina (Syndrome X)
    Female > Male

Mitral Regurgitation
    Male > Female
    Males are more likely to have abnormal leaflet.

Mitral Stenosis
    Female > Male
    Females are more likely to have rheumatic mitral stenosis.

Females have longer post-surgical survival and better functional improvements after surgery for mitral stenosis.

Mitral Stenosis — Rheumatic
    Female > Male (2:1)

Mitral Valve Disease
    Female > Male

Mitral Valve Prolapse
    Female > Male (2:1)
        Under age 20 years
    Female = Male
        After age 20 years, but males are more severely affected than females after age 50 years.
    Severe regurgitation develops more often in males. The risk of developing infective endocarditis is also higher in males with MVP.
    Females live longer than men do before mitral insufficiency develops and symptomatic coronary artery disease develops at a later age in females.
    Severe complications with mitral valve prolapse:
        Male > Female
            Severe Mitral Regurgitation: Male > Female 2:1
            Endocarditis: Male > Female
        Males are 2 times more likely to require surgery for MVP after age 50 years than females.

Myocardial Infarction
    Male > Female
        Age 40–70 years
    Male = Female
        Age over 70 years
    Females experience more lethal (1.2–1.7:1) and severe first acute MI. 42% of women who have MI die within 1 year compared to 10–24% of men. Within 6 yrs of an MI, 21% of men and 33% of women will have a recurrent MI.
    The 4-year postinfarction mortality for women is 36% compared to 21% for men. Also women that survive have a higher infarct recurrence rate and more likely to have recurrent angina than men. Women may not be treated as aggressively as men for various reasons.

Women have higher rates of depression after an MI.

Women have a greater likelihood of unstable angina as the initial manifestations of acute cardiac ischemia and less extensive coronary narrowing at the time of the acute ischemic episode.

Women are less likely to have chest pain at presentation of MI than men (38% vs. 49%).

The ISIS-2 study showed that women have a higher mortality following thrombolytic therapy than men.

Women that are at high risk when they undergo CABG have higher operative mortality, lower short and long term graft patency rates, and less relief of angina. Some possible reasons include smaller coronary vessels in women, older age, more frequent comorbid conditions and more advanced coronary disease at referral.

Women tend to have more complications including vessel dissection after percutaneous transluminal coronary angioplasty than men.

Silent and unrecognized MIs are more common in females.

Females with MI have a higher complication and mortality rate than men.

Females receiving antithrombolytic treatment have a higher risk of hemorrhagic and total strokes.

Mortality for MI in females receiving thrombolytics is greater than for men.

After MI, females have more CHF at a higher ejection fraction than men.

Lack of social support after MI increases the 6–12 month mortality rate more in males than females.

Females are more likely to have cardiac rupture after an MI.

Females have a higher ejection fraction post MI than males.

Congestive heart failure complicating MI is more common in females.

Females with coronary artery disease seem to have more diabetes mellitus, hypertension and elevated cholesterol compared to men.

Males are more likely to present with MI as initial presentation of coronary heart disease, however, a MI as the initial manifestation of CHD is more likely fatal in females.

Females tend to have less ST segment elevation, more non-Q wave infarcts, and more atypical symptoms. Females with MI are more likely to have nausea, vomiting, abdominal pain, fatigue, dyspnea, shoulder and neck pain, and palpitations, but are less likely to report diaphorisis than males.

Females have higher rate of reinfarction at 1–2 years post MI.

Females have higher rates of mitral valve rupture after MI.

Females have higher rates of post MI strokes.

Coronary plaques in females have more cellularity and fibrous tissue. Females tend to have higher fibrinogen and Factor VIII levels.

Females have more noncoronary chest pain syndromes.

Females are less likely to smoke than males.

Females tend to have more serious presentation with increased prevalence of tachycardia, rales, heart block and higher Killip class on presentation. Still, females are less likely to receive thrombolytics, or receive it later, and are less likely to be admitted to coronary care unit and are less likely to undergo diagnostic catherization during their hospital stay than men with MI.

Women have higher rates of in-hospital complications from MI including bleeding, stroke, shock, myocardial rupture, and recurrent angina than do men, although most differences disappear when corrected for age and comorbidity.

Males have a higher rate of prehospital sudden death.

Females are at increased risk of intracranial hemorrhage from use of thrombolytic therapy for MI (1.59 vs. 1.0).

Elevated levels of Factor VIIa are associated with increased risk of recurrent cardiac events in postinfarct women but not men.

D-dimer is more predictive for cardiac events in postinfarct men than women.

Myxomas
    Female > Male (7:3)
    36% occur in the left atrium.

Nonrheumatic Aortic Valve Disease
    Aortic Stenosis of Bicuspid Aortic Valve
        Male > Female to develop complications
    Aortic Insufficiency
        In females, usually due to bicuspid aortic valve
        In males—idiopathic aortic root dilation

Nonrheumatic Mitral Valve Disease
    Female > Male (2:1)
        Mitral Annular Calcification

Female > Male
: Systemic Lupus Erythematosus
  Libman-Sacks vegetations

Obesity
: Black Female > White Females   Black Males ≅ White Males
     50%   30–35%   30%   30–35%
  Increased in black females, Hispanics and Pacific Islanders.

Orthostatic Hypotension
: Increased risk of vascular death in elderly males.

Orthostatic Intolerance
: Female > Male
  Usually between 20–50 years old.

Palpitations
: The occurrence is often noticed to increase in the luteal phase of the menstrual cycle in females taking oral contraceptives with high estrogen content.

Patent Ductus Arteriosus
: Female > Male (2–3:1)

Pericardial Disease in the Vasculitis/Connective Tissue Group
: Male > Female
    Overall (although females usually have higher predominance of connective tissue disease)
    Rheumatoid Arthritis (Male > Female)
      Patients usually have high rheumatoid factor titers.
    Systemic Lupus Erythematosus
      Males are overrepresented and are more likely to develop constriction of the pericardium.
    Seronegative Spondyloarthropathies (Male > Female)
    Takayasu's Arteritis (Female > Male)

Pericarditis
: Male > Female

Periodic Paralysis
: Male > Female
  People are at increased risk of ventricular tachycardia.

Cardiology

Peripheral Arterial Disease
> Male > Female (1.27:1)
> Hypertension increases risk of claudication 2.5 times in men and 4 times in women.
> Intermittent Claudication
>> Male > Female
>> Males report more symptoms, but no difference seen on objective testing. Men receive more procedures for symptoms than women.
>> Among male smokers, the risk of peripheral artery disease (PAD) is increased with packs per years smoked, and depth of inhalation, but decreases with more exercise (not seen in women).
>> Lipoprotein A level is risk factor for developing PAD in women, but not in men.
>> Diabetes has more influence on the development of PAD in females.
>> Although women develop peripheral artery disease, they rarely develop Buerger's disease.

Pheochromocytoma
> Female > Male

Polyarteritis Nodosa
> Male > Female (2.5:1)

Popliteal Artery Aneurysm
> Male > Female

Popliteal Artery Entrapment Syndrome
> Male > Female

Postural Tachycardia Syndrome
> Female > Male
> Primarily occurs in young women.

Primary Lymphedema
> Female > Male

Primary Pulmonary Hypertension
> Female > Male (4:1)
> Sporadic and familial forms
> Fewer males are born in PPH families than in the population at large, suggesting that the PPH gene may influence fertilization or cause male fetal wastage.

Prinzmetal's Angina
> Male > Female
> Patients with this are usually younger than patients with typical angina due to atherosclerosis.

Pulmonary Artery Sarcoma
> Female > Male (2:1)

Raynauds Phenomenon
> Female > Male (2:1)
>> 1° Raynauds
>>> Females are 60–90% of cases.
>> 2° Raynauds
>>> Less sex differences noted.

Recurrent Venous Thrombosis
> Male > Female

Renovascular Hypertension
> Male > Female (2:1)
>> Atherosclerosis
>> Accounts for 90% of cases. As age increases the sex distribution comes more equal.
> Female > Male (8:1)
>> Fibromuscular dysplasia
>> Usually in younger females.

Rheumatic Cardiac Regurgitation
> Male > Female (3:1)

Rheumatic Mitral Regurgitation
> Male > Female (1.5:1)

Rheumatic Mitral Valve Stenosis
> Female > Male (2–3:1)
> Females are more likely to progress to severe mitral stenosis; however the prognosis is worse for males.

Males tend to develop more calcification of the mitral valve.
Females are more likely to have nonfatal and fatal arterial emboli.

Small Aorta Syndrome
Female > Male
Seen exclusively in females of small stature, heavy smokers and often have high cholesterol levels.

Smoking
Males > Female
Rate of decline in smoking is less in females.

Spenic Artery Aneurysm
Female > Male (4:1)

Spontaneous Coronary Dissection
Female > Male (3:1)

Stroke
Male > Female (1.3:1)
Males with LVH have 6–10 fold increased risk of stroke than males without LVH. Females with LVH have 3–5 times higher risk of stroke than females without LVH.
Occurrence of carotid artery plaques is greater in males than females except after age 80 years.

Subclavian Steal Syndrome
Male > Female (2:1)
Males affected at younger age on average than females.

Sudden Cardiac Death Syndrome
Male > Female (3.8:1)
A manifestation of coronary heart disease, especially in males.
Sudden death without a history of coronary artery disease appears more common in females (63% vs. 44%).
LVH on EKG is a strong predictor of sudden cardiac death in males but only modestly in females.
In chronic coronary artery disease, risk is two times as likely in males.
Complex ventricular ectopy after MI has a worse prognosis for men.
Incidence of sudden death in females lags behind males by 20 years.

Sudden death rate of females was only 32% of males' sudden death rate even after symptomatic myocardial infarct, despite similar or increased overall mortality rate in females.

Predictors of sudden death in males include: smoking, glucose intolerance, cholesterol level, hypertension, left ventricular hypertrophy, and PVCs. Predictors in females include: smoking, hypertension and psychosocial factors.

Sudden Death in Competitive Athletes
Male > Female (9:1)

Superior Mesenteric Artery Syndrome
Female > Male (2:1)

Superior Vena Cava Syndrome
Male > Female

Sustained Bradycardia
Male > Female (3:1)

Syndrome-X
Female > Male

Systemic Lupus Erythematosus
Female > Male (9–10:1)

Females with SLE are 50 times more likely to experience myocardial infarction than females without SLE.

Pericarditis is occasionally seen.

Takayasu's Arteritis
Female > Male (6–9:1)

Primarily in females, around 40 years old, and from East Asia.

Tetralogy of Fallot
Male > Female (slightly)

Thoracic Aortic Aneurysm
Male > Female (age-adjusted rates)

Incidence is increasing in females, especially in elderly females.

The probability of rupture: Female > Male (33% Female, 9% Male).

Probability of elective repair: 25% Male, 13% Female.

In one large study, females appeared to have more descending aneurysms (2:1) while males had more ascending (2:1) aneurysms, but the rupture rate was 3 times higher in the descending aneurysms.

Thoracic Artery Aneurysm
    Male > Female (2:1)

Thoracic Outlet Syndrome
    Male = Female
        Arterial Type
    Male > Female
        Venous Type
    Female > Male (3.5:1)
        Neurologic Type

Thromboangiitis Obliterans
    Male > Female (3:1)
    Primarily in young male smokers, however increasing in females.

Thrombophlebitis, Superficial
    Male = Female
        Suppurative
    Female > Male (2:1)
        Mondor's
    Female > Male
        Thromboangiitis Obliterans (males are 1–19% of cases)

Thrombosis, Deep Venous
    Female > Male (1.2:1)

Torsade de Pointes-Drug Induced or Bradyarrhythmia Induced
    Female > Male (7:3)

Tricuspid Stenosis
    Female > Male

Turner's Syndrome
    Females only
    Aortic Coarctation is common.

Unstable Angina
    Female > Male
    Unstable angina/non-ST segment elevation MI's are more common in females.
    Females are more likely to fail percutaneous coronary interventions.
    CABG in females—mortality 3.9% vs. 2.3% in men.

Perioperative morbidity for MI, respiratory failure and stroke is also higher in females. A high incidence of sternal infections occurs in females and may be due to obesity. Females tend to have more comorbid conditions preoperatively and have more diffuse coronary disease and left ventricle dysfunction. Females also tend to have smaller distal vessels (as a function of smaller body surface area).

Valvular Aortic Stenosis
   Male > Female
   Females more frequently exhibit normal or even supranormal ventricular performance and a smaller, thicker-walled concentric hypertrophied left ventricle with diastolic dysfunction. Men more frequently have eccentric left ventricular hypertrophy, excessive systolic wall stress, systolic dysfunction and ventricular dilatation. Females undergoing aortic valve replacement and CABG have higher perioperative mortality rates.
   In patients undergoing aortic stenosis surgery, the myocardium of the female presents fewer modifications in the collagen structure.
   For the same decrease in the orifice of the aortic valve, females undergoing surgery have a larger increase in the LV wall thickness, an increased echocardiographic shortening fraction and increased ejection fraction.

Valvular Heart Disease
   Acquired Valvular Heart Disease

Mitral Stenosis:	Female > Male (7–8:3)
Mitral Regurgitation:	Male > Female (34–47% are female)
Mitral Valve Prolapse:	Female > Male (3:1)
Aortic Stenosis:	Male > Female (3:1)
Aortic Regurgitation:	Male > Female (4:1)
Truspid Stenosis:	Female > Male (9:1) Almost always associated with mitral stenosis
Coarctation of Aorta:	Male > Female

In elderly patients, valvular disease is seen in Female > Male, probably due to longer lifespan of women.

Females are hospitalized more than males for valvular heart disease and have more valvular surgery. 60% of heart valve replacements are in women.

Complication and mortality rates in nonrheumatic valvular heart disease are higher in men.

Rheumatic Valve Disease
> Female > Male (1.2–1.5:1)
> Susceptibility to acute rheumatic fever in childhood and teenage years:
> > White Male > White Female (2–3:1)
> > No gender differences noted in nonwhites

Acute Rheumatic Fever—manifestations are similar, except females may develop pure chorea or chronic rheumatic heart disease without other acute signs of illness.

Acute Rheumatic Heart Disease Mortality
> Females > Males by 30% despite the lower incidence of rheumatic fever in females.

In rheumatic heart disease, mitral valve disorders are 2.3 times higher in females, while aortic valve disorders are 3.6 times higher in males.

Chronic rheumatic heart disease mortality is two times greater in females.

Stenosing calcification of the mitral ring in mitral stenosis is more common in females.

Variant Angina
> Female > Male

Varicose Veins
> Female > Male (2–5:1)

Ventricular Arrhythmias
> Premature ventricular contractions (PVCs) and brief runs of nonsustained ventricular tachycardia are more common in males (10% vs. 4%).
>
> The relationship between PVCs and nonsustained ventricular tachycardia is less significant for females than males. In males with coronary artery disease, frequent PVCs or complex arrhythmias are associated with increased risk of mortality and myocardial infarction but this is not seen in females.

Ventricular Septal Defect
> Male ≅ Female
> But Male > Female if secondary to myocardial infarction

Viral Pericarditis
> Male > Female (3–4:1)

White Coat Hypertension
    Female > Male

Wolff-Parkinson White Syndrome
    Male > Female

Pulmonology

Anatomy and Physiology

The adult lung weighs 850 grams in males, 750 grams in females. In females, pulmonary capacity is less, absolutely and proportionately, the sternum being shorter, the thoracic inlet more oblique and the suprasternal notch level at the third thoracic vertebra (second in males). The upper ribs are more mobile in females, allowing greater upper thoracic expansion. The female clavicle is shorter, thinner, less curved smoother and its acromial end carried lower than the sternal. In males it is level with or slightly above the sternal end when the arm is pendent. Boys have smaller airways for a given lung size than girls. Boys 4–6 years of age have also been found to have lower flow rates and higher airways resistance compared to girls the same age. Type I and Type II muscle fibers of the respiratory muscles are of larger diameter in males.

The respiratory capacity of females fluctuates according to the cyclical variations of their sex hormones: before the onset of periods, women's airways become slightly narrower, which requires more ventilation. The ventilatory requirements are 30% greater during the luteal phase than during the follicular phase of the menstrual cycle.

Normal men appear to be more vulnerable to load induced hypoventilation than women due to increased collapse of the upper airway. Men develop more severe hypopnea in response to identical applied external loads. Sensitivity to transient hypercapnia and its interaction with hyperoxia are weaker in women than men.

Females have greater minute ventilations and lower tidal volumes than males. The ventilatory response to high carbon dioxide levels is greater in males. Women have higher ventilatory responses in the luteal phase than in the follicular phase of the menstrual cycle.

There is an inverse association of the waist-hip ratio (WHR) with

FEV1 in men but not in women. Larger values of WHR are associated with greater reductions in FVC in men compared to women.

Men have a higher resting ventilation and metabolic rate than women. Women have higher VE/VCO_2 than men and lower resting end-title PCO_2.

Normal Predicted Average Peak Flow (liters/min)

Age	Male Height (inches)					Female Height (inches)				
	60	65	70	75	80	55	60	65	70	75
15	511	531	548	564	578	423	438	451	453	473
20	554	575	594	611	626	444	460	474	486	497
25	580	603	622	640	656	455	471	485	497	509
30	594	617	637	655	672	458	474	489	502	513
35	599	622	643	661	677	458	474	488	501	512
40	597	620	641	659	675	453	469	483	496	507
45	591	613	633	651	668	446	462	474	488	499
50	580	602	622	640	656	437	453	466	478	489
55	566	588	608	625	640	427	442	455	467	477
60	551	572	591	607	622	415	430	443	454	464
65	533	554	572	588	603	403	417	430	441	451
70	515	535	552	568	582	390	414	416	427	436
75	496	515	532	547	560	377	391	402	413	422

Human Inhalation Rates for Men and Women By Activity Level (m^3/hour)

	Resting	Light	Moderate	Heavy
Adult Male	0.7	0.8	2.5	4.8
Adult Female	0.3	0.5	1.6	2.9

Diseases

Adenocarcinoma of the Lung
    Female > Male
    Occurs in both smokers and nonsmokers.
    Most develop peripherally in the lung.

Adenoid Cystic Carcinoma of Lung
    Female > Male (slightly)

Adult Respiratory Distress Syndrome
    Mortality rate is almost twice as great in males compared to females.
    Mortality in blacks is greater than whites.

Alpha-1 Antitrypsin Deficiency
    Female > Male
    Smoking significantly worsens the disease.

Arterial Gas Embolism
    Male > Female
    Usually associated with SCUBA diving.

Asbestosis
    Male > Female

Asthma
    Male > Female
        Under 10 years of age
        The pulmonary system of young girls (< 4 years old) performs better because of greater expiratory flow and greater ability to relax after a deep breath.
        In male children, a history of asthma is associated with a larger decrease in midexpiratory flow and forced expiratory flow at 75% of expired FVC than in female children with history of asthma.
    Males = Females
        Puberty
    Female > Male
        Adult (2:1)
        The predominance of disease in adult women is believed related to hormones. Up to 40% of females note an increase of asthma symptoms perimenstrually. The perimenstrual interval, defined as day 26–4 of the cycle, is the most common time for women to go to the emergency room for asthma attacks.
        At menopause the risk of developing asthma is again reduced.
        From 1982–1992 the prevalence of asthma in females rose 82% compared to 29% in males, and females had twice the death rate as males. Women may have more severe disease and more asthma triggers and symptoms.

Hospitalization incidence for asthma is higher in male children (2:1) but becomes greater in females in the 20–50 year age group.

Women with asthma appear to have a lower quality of life than males with asthma.

Men are less likely to report severe asthma symptoms and activity limitation than women at similar levels of obstruction.

Blastomycosis
    Male > Female

Bronchial Responsiveness
    Female > Male
        After puberty

Bronchiolitis
    Male > Female

Carcinosarcoma
    Male > Female

Carney's Triad
    Female > Male
    This is a syndrome of pulmonary chondroma, extrarenal paraganglioma, and gastric epithelioid leiomyosarcoma.

Central Alveolar Hypoventilation
    Male > Female

Chlamydia Pneumoniae
    Male > Female (10–25% more)

Chondroma of Mediastinum
    Male > Female (2:1)

Chronic Eosinophilic Pneumonia
    Male > Female (2:1)

Chronic Granulomatous Disease
    Male > Female
    60% are X-linked.

Chronic Mountain Sickness
    Male > Female

Chronic Obstuctive Pulmonary Disease
    Male > Female (2.3:1)

Congenital Bronchogenic Cyst
    Male > Female
    Occurs more frequently on the right side.

Congenital Cystic Disease of Lung-Diffuse
    Male > Female (2:1)

Congenital Diaphragmatic Hernia
    Male > Female (2:1)

Congenital Lobar Emphysema
    Male > Female

Cor Pulmonale
    Male > Female

Costochondritis
    Female > Male
        Predominantly female

Coumarin-Induced Skin Necrosis
    Female > Male

Croup
    Male > Female

Cystic Fibrosis
    Male = Female
    Although the frequency of occurrence is the same, males live slightly longer than females by a median of 4 years.
    77% of males and 82% of females with CF die of lung disease.
    The mortality of CF in the first year of life is higher in males but male advantage becomes obvious after infancy.
    Asthma, bronchopulmonary dysplasia and other airways diseases tend to be more severe in boys than in girls in the first six years of life probably due to the relatively smaller airways size in boys during these early years.
    Males have more reproductive difficulties and boys with CF have antibodies to sperm.
    Men with cystic fibrosis are sterile because of azoospermic absence of vas deferens.

Females with CF have delayed onset of menarche.
The rate of decline of pulmonary function is more in girls than boys with CF.
Girls have better acceleration of growth and better weight for height than boys.
Girls have a greater decline in FEV1 after colonization with the bacteria *Bordetella cepacia* and are colonized with *Psuedomonas aeruginosa* about 1 year earlier than males.

Desmoid Tumor of the Chest Wall
  Female > Male

Drowning and Near Drowning
  Male > Female (4:1)
  Risk taking in males and alcohol use contributes to this difference.

Drug Induced Lupus Erythematosus
  Female > Male

Eosinophilic Granuloma of Chest Wall
  Male > Female

Eosinophilic Granulomatosis
  Male > Female (slightly)
  More than 90% are smokers and almost exclusively occurs in whites.

Eosinophilic Pneumonia
  Male ≥ Female
  Usually in 4th decade in male, 6th decade in female.

Epiglottitis
  Male > Female

Epithelioid Hemangioendothelioma
  Female > Male (4:1)

Ewing's Sarcoma of Chest Wall
  Male > Female

Farmer's Lung Disease
  Male > Female

Fetal Lung Immaturity
    Male > Female
    White > Black

Germ Cell Tumor of the Mediastinum
    Male > Female

Goodpasture's Syndrome
    Male > Female (7:1)
    This is the classic form. The average age of onset is 27 years. There is a form of glomerulonephritis alone that occurs primarily in elderly females.

Hamartoma of the Lung
    Male > Female (2:1)

Hiccups, Persistent
    Male > Female

Hughes-Stoven Syndrome
    Male > Female

Hyperventilation Syndrome
    Female > Male (2–7:1)

Idiopathic Hypereosinophilic Syndrome
    Male > Female

Idiopathic Pulmonary Fibrosis
    Male > Female (slightly)
    In one study the prevalence was 20 per 100,000 in men and 13 per 100,000 in women.
    Females tend to live longer.

Idiopathic Rapidly Progressive Glomerulonephritis
    Male > Female (2:1)
    20–50% have lung involvement with alveolar hemorrhage.

Intrathoracic Goiter
    Female > Male

Langerhan's Cell Histiocytosis
    Male > Female (slightly)

Laryngeal Cancer
    Male > Female (5:1)

Lipoma of Bronchus
    Male > Female

Loeffler's Syndrome
    Female > Male
    Usually middle-age white female with history of asthma.

Lower Repiratory Infections in Children
    Male > Female

Lung Abscess
    Male > Female (4:1)

Lung Cancer
    Male > Female
    Lung cancer is responsible for > 30% of cancer deaths in males, > 25% in females.
    Tobacco smoking is implicated in 85% of cases. Women are likely to develop lung cancer after less smoking and much earlier in life, regardless of their smoking history. Greater expression of the gastrin-releasing-peptide receptor in females may explain this difference.
    Polymorphisms in CYP1A1 and glutathione S-transferase M1 contribute to an increased risk of lung cancer in females.

Lymphangioleiomyomatosis
    Female only

Lymphoblastic Nonhodgkins Lymphoma
    Male > Female (2–4:1)

Lymphomatoid Granulomatosis
    Male > Female (slightly)

Malignant Fibrous Histiocytoma of the Lung
    Male > Female

Mediastinal Carcinoid Tumor
    Male > Female

Mediastinal Thyroid Tumor
    Female > Male

Mycobacterium Avium-Intracelluare Complex Disease
    Male = Female
        With underlying lung disease

Female > Male (4:1)
  : Without underlying lung disease
  Male > Female (9:1)
  : With immune deficiency disease—with HIV
  Male > Female (2:1)
  : With immune deficiency disease—without HIV

Mycobacterium Chelonei
: Female > Male

Mycobacterium Fortuitum
: Male > Female

Microscopic Polyangiitis
: Male > Female—(slightly)
  Pulmonary hemorrhage is seen in 12–19% of cases.

Nasal Polyps
: Male > Female (2:1)

Necrotizing Sarcoid Granulomatosis
: Female > Male

Nonseminoma Germ Cell Tumor of the Mediastinum
: Male > Female

Oculocutaneous Albinism
: Female = Male
  But lung disease (fibrosis) is twice as high in females.

Osteochondroma of Chest Wall
: Male > Female

Osteoid Osteoma of Chest Wall
: Male > Female

Pancoast Tumor
: Male > Female

Paracoccidioidomycosis
: Male > Female (9:1)
  Skin test results demonstrate a 50:50 relationship between men and women, although clinical disease is more common in men.

Pectus Carinatum
: Male > Female (4:1)

Pectus Excavatum
    Male > Female (3–4:1)

Pigeon Breeder's Disease
    Male > Female
    However in Mexico, Female > Male because of differing patterns of exposure.

Pleural Mesothelioma-Malignant
    Male > Female (3–4:1)

Pneumocystis Carinii Pneumonia
    Male > Female
    Reflects HIV prevalence

Pneumonia, Bacterial
    Male > Female
    Mortality greater in elderly males than elderly females.

Pneumonia, Mycoplasma
    Male > Female

Pneumonia, Viral
    Male = Female
    But male sex may predispose to more severe disease in respiratory syncytial virus infections.

Pneumothorax
    Male > Female (6:1)
    Primary Spontaneous Pneumothorax
        Male cases—7.4-18 cases per 100 thousand
        Female cases—1.2-6 cases per 100 thousand
        Smoking increases the risk 22 times for males and 8 times for females.
    Secondary Spontaneous Pneumothorax
        Male cases—6.3 per 100 thousand
        Female cases—2 per 100 thousand

Primary Cancer of the Mediastinum
    Male > Female

Primary Pulmonary Hypertension
    Female > Male (1.7–3:1)

Primary Pulmonary Lymphoma
   Male > Female (slightly)

Primary Spontaneous Pneumothorax
   Male > Female (3–6:1)
   Typically in tall, thin boys between 10–30 years of age.
   Smoking increases the risk up to 20 fold in men.

Pulmonary Alveolar Proteinosis
   Male > Female (2–4:1)

Pulmonary Chemodectoma
   Female > Male (4:1)

Pulmonary Embolism
   Female > Male (3:2)
   Increased incidence of death in women.

Pulmonary Hypertension Associated with Connective Tissue Disease
   Female > Male

Pulmonary Sequestration
   Male > Female (4:1)
      Extralobar
   Female = Male
      Intralobar

Respiratory Distress Syndrome, Neonate
   Male ≥ Female
   Usually more severe in males and males have worse outcome at any birth weight and gestational age.
   The lungs of female fetuses are about 1 week more mature than males. Estrogen stimulates fetal lung surfactant synthesis and testosterone may inhibit surfactant production, making males more likely to get RDS.
   Male fetuses are exposed to higher levels of Mullerian inhibiting substance (MIS) and recent evidence indicates MIS may inhibit lung development.

Respiratory Syncytial Virus Infection
   Male = Female
      Outpatient
   Male > Female (2:1)
      Hospitalized

Rheumatoid Arthritis-Associated Interstitial Lung Disease
> Male > Female
> Although, females have more rheumatoid arthritis.

Rheumatoid Lung Disease
> Male > Female
> Rheumatoid arthritis is more common in females
> Bronchiolitis obliterans is more common in females than males with rheumatoid arthritis.
> Pleural involvement in patients with RA occurs in 24% of males and 16% of females.
> Necrobiotic rheumatoid nodules are more common in males.
> Interstitial lung disease is more common in men.

Rheumatoid Pleurisy
> Male > Female

Sarcoidosis
> Female > Male (8:1)
> Black > White

Sarcoidosis: Granulomatous Skin Lesions
> Female > Male
>> Acute Myopathy
> Female > Male
>> Acute Polyathritiis

Sclerosing Hemangioma of the Lung
> Female > Male (4:1)

Scoliosis
> Female > Male (4:1)
>> Overall
> Male > Female (3:2)
>> Infant onset
>> Infantile scoliosis usually involves a curvature to the left.
> Female > Male (9:1)
>> Adolescent onset
>> Scoliosis in adolescent girls is usually rightwards.

Seminoma
> Male > Female

Silicosis
    Male > Female

Sjogren's Syndrome
    Female > Male
    However severe restrictive lung disease more likely to occur in black men with cardiac involvement also noted.

Sleep Apnea, Obstructive
    Male > Female (8:1)
        Adults
        Men are more likely to snore, to stop breathing during sleep, and to report drowsy driving; whereas women more likely to feel tired after sleep or during wake time.
    Male = Female
        Prepubertal

Small Cell Lung Cancer
    Male = Female
    Female sex carries a worse prognosis.

Snoring
    Male > Female
    45% of males and 30% of females over 65 years of age snore.
    Increased blood pressure is two times greater in snorers.

Solitary Plasmocytoma of Chest Wall
    Male > Female

Spontaneous Hemopneumothorax
    Male > Female
    Only 0.2% of women with spontaneous pneumothorax develop blood in the pleural space compared to 3–12% of males.

Squamous Cell Cancer of the Lung
    Male > Female
    Occurs primarily in cigarette smokers.
    Most develop acentrally.

Systemic Sclerosis
    Female > Male
    Restrictive lung disease is more common in males.

Takayasu's Arteritis
    Female > Male (6–9:1)

Thoracic Outlet Syndrome
    Female > Male

Thymic Large B-Cell Lymphoma
    Female > Male (slightly)

Tracheitis, Bacterial
    Male > Female (1.8:1)

Transient Tachpynea of Newborn
    Male > Female

Tuberculosis
    Male > Female
    Reflects male predominance in AIDS, shelters, and prisons.

Tuberous Sclerosis
    Female = Male
    But females are more likely to develop pulmonary disease.

Wegener's Granulomatosis
    Male > Female (2–3:1–2)

X-linked Agammaglobulinemia
    Male > Female

Yellow Nail Syndrome
    Female > Male (1.6:1)

Endocrinology/Metabolism

Anatomy and Physiology

The pituitary gland in females is larger than in males, and increases in size during pregnancy. There are more lactotrope cells in the pituitary gland of females. The number of lactrope cells in the pars distalis is greater in females. Females have more large sized secretory granules and males have more small sized secretory granules in the gonadotrope cells of the pituitary gland. Brain nuclei that exhibit sexual dimorphism in humans include the sexually dimorphic nucleus of the hypothalamus, the anterior commissure, and the bed nuclei of the stria terminalis. An empty sella may be found in 18% of normal women. The bed nucleus of the stria terminalis in the hypothalamus is larger in males.

The production rate of lutenizing hormone is higher in men than ovulating women but the postmenopausal female has the highest production rate. The male pituitary secretes both FSH and LH in a pulsatile but generally constant and sustained manner but the female pituitary secretion of LH and FSH is cyclic and is characterized by a preovulatory gonadotropin surge that leads to ovulation. The mean FSH and LH content of the fetal pituitary gland is higher in females. At birth the LH level abruptly increases in male neonates, but not females. LH pulses are higher in male infants. By 6 months of age in males and 2–3 yrs of age in females, the levels of plasma gonadotropins decrease to low values until the time of puberty. In men, the pulsatile release of LH has a periodicity of about 90–120 minutes and precedes testosterone secretion by 40 minutes. In women, LH pulse frequency and amplitude vary during the menstrual cycle from 1 pulse/hr in the midfollicular phase to 1 pulse/5 hr in the late luteal phase. The FSH pulse amplitude and FSH response to LHRH is greater in female infants. Short term estrogen administration in men does not sensitize the pituitary to LHRH as estrogen does in women. From late fetal age through puberty, FSH stimulates aromatase and estrogen synthesis by the ovary. Whereas in boys, estrogen synthesis is not detectable in fetal or prepubertal Leydig cells and is at a very low level until LH stimulates Leydig cell aromatase at late stage 2 or stage 3 of male secondary maturation. During puberty, the urinary FSH level rises 5 times in boys and girls but the urinary LH level increases 50 times in boys and 100 times in girls. Estradiol levels are higher in prepubertal girls than boys. Prepubertal girls and boys have similar testosterone levels except during the first 3–5 months of male infancy where prepubertal levels are found.

Premenopausal females have higher growth hormone production rates than young men. Serum growth hormone level rises during pubertal development and the rise starts at a chronologic earlier age in females. Increased growth hormone secretion and serum IGF-1 levels occur earlier in girls than boys during pubertal development. Insulin Growth Factor I (IGF-1) levels are higher in females and peak at an earlier age in females. Men tend to have higher insulin levels and insulin resistance than females but gender differences decrease with age. Growth hormone secretion is greater in women than men despite similar reference ranges of serum insulin-like growth factor 1 in adult men and women. The mass of GH secreted per burst is greater in females but the orderliness of the 24-hour GH release process is less orderly in females. Males are more responsive than females to exogenous growth hormone administration. Interleukin-6 plays an important role in pituitary and peripheral hormone secretion in women only.

Pubertal growth occurs earlier in girls but is 3 to 5 centimeters greater in magnitude in boys. Girls on average experience their first menstrual period at age 13 years and reach their adult height by age 15 years. Girls generally grow 2–2.5 additional inches after menarche. In males, the testicles enlarge at puberty and adult height may not be reached until age 20–21 years. Large increases in muscle mass occur in males between 16–21 years. Sex related difference in adult height is about 13 cm due to earlier cessation of growth in females. The ratio of sitting height to standing height is higher in pubertal and adult females than males. Shoulder width is greater in boys while hips enlarge more in girls and the pelvic inlet widens in females at puberty. At puberty the mandible and nose enlarge more in boys. Axillary Hair: Appears about age 14 years in boys and most girls have axillary hair by age 12 years. Skeletal maturation is more advanced in girls than boys of the same age. The total bone mineral density is greater in males by the late teenage years. (Peaks at age 15.8 years in females and 17.5 years in males). Lean body mass, skeletal mass, and body fat are equal in prepubertal boys and girls, but mature men have 1.5 times the lean body mass and almost 1.5 times the skeletal mass of mature women. Mature females have two times as much body fat as men. The increase in lean body mass starts at age 6 years in females and 9.5 years in males.

Overweight is defined as a BMI of 27.8 or more in men and 27.3 or more in women. Severe overweight is defined as a BMI of 31.1 or more in men and 32.3 or more in women. Males tend to have more abdominal fat but less femoral-gluteal fat as compared to females. Adult female of same height and weight as adult males have a lower basal metabolism and lower energy expenditure per unit of work. Under conditions of moderate exercise, females primarily use fatty acids, sparing muscle glycogen reserves and permitting sustained performance. Females have a greater potential for oxidative metabolism in their muscles. Within the abdominal area, females have more lipolytic activity in subcutaneous fat whereas males show more lipolytic activity in visceral fat. These differences disappear after menopause. Visual distribution of fat in boys (central or apple shaped: android) is different than in females (pear shaped: gynoid) The nadir of the curve of body mass index and mortality is 23.5–24.9 years for men and 22.0–23.4 years for women. Fat content is higher in females than males. There is a gradual overall increase in fat content until the 6–7th decade of life. Females are more efficient at utilizing fat calories than men. Females have a tendency to metabolize fat instead of carbohydrates during exercise.

Men have more muscle cells and greater size of individual muscle cells than women. Muscle mass is 54% of body weight in adolescent boys and 42% of body weight of adolescent girls. At puberty, with the change in fat composition, body water increases 5% in men and decreases 5% in women. Intracellular H_2O increases at puberty in boys from 36 to 39% and decreases in girls from 36 to 29%. Among adults 25–44 years of age, the body weight, measured at 10 year intervals, increased by an average of 3.4% in men and 5.2% in women in the first National Health and Nutrition Examination Survey.

Formula to calculate body mass index using weight and height
    Men: % Fat = 1.218 (W/H^2)–10.13
    Women: % Fat = 1.48 (W/H^2)–7.17
    BMI of 25 is considered upper limit of normal

Waist/Hip ratio: > 0.72 is abnormal but complication rates increase substantially at ratios > 1 for men and 0.9 for women.

A Waist-to-Hip ratio of > 1.0 for men and > 0.8 for women is associated with an increased coronary heart disease risk.

Testosterone

In males, most produced in testes.

In females, 2/3 produced in adrenals.

In females, testosterone is associated with higher adipose tissue lipoprotein lipase and larger abdominal fat cells. In contrast, testosterone tends to be lower in men with more visceral fat.

In males, the testes produce only 15–20% of total body production of estradiol whereas most plasma estradiol in females is produced by the ovaries. Testosterone binding globulin (TBG) level: The prepubertal levels are similar in boys and girls. After puberty, levels increase in boys. Plasma free testosterone level is 40 times higher in men than women. Insulin decreases TBG levels in men and low levels of TBG predict the development of Type 2 diabetes in men.

Manual stimulation of the breast causes ≥ 2 times increase in prolactin levels in 1/3 of women but there is no response in men. The prolactin level is similar in boys and girls (4.0 vs. 4.5 ug/L) prepuberty, but adult female levels are usually higher than in males (8.3 vs. 5.2 ug/L).

Serum leptin levels are higher in females by 2–3 times. Women have more subcutaneous fat that secretes more leptin. Leptin mRNA expression and secretion are higher in adipocytes from females. Leptin levels are higher in obese girls than obese boys.

Rise in leptin levels occurs about 1 year earlier in girls than boys. The level of leptin peaks at Tanner genital stage 2 in boys and Tanner breast stage 5 in girls. Enlargement of adipose cells after menopause is more gradual in men and more abrupt in women.

Response of TSH to TRH is greater in females than males, especially in females over age 40 years. Elderly males reveal diminished TSH response to TRH injection relative to elderly females. Estrogen appears to enhance the response to TRH. Nuclear androgen receptor content is higher in normal thyroid tissue of males than females. Thyroxine binding globulin levels are slightly higher in females than males. Thyroglobulin concentration is higher in females. Basal metabolic rate: the basal oxygen consumption is higher in males than females. Antibodies to thyroglobulin and thyroid peroxidase in the general population are 5 times more common in females.

Mean value for Cholesterol and Triglyceride Levels

Male (years)	Cholesterol (mg/dl)	Triglyceride (mg/dl)
0–10	160	55
10–20	155	70
20–30	175	110
30–39	195	135
40–49	210	150
50–59	215	145
60–69	215	140
70+	205	130
Female (years)		
0–10	160	60
10–20	160	75
20–30	165	75
30–39	180	85
40–49	200	100
50–59	225	120
60–69	230	130
70+	230	130

At all ages women have higher levels of high-density lipoprotein cholesterol and levels are only minimally changed by menopause. In contrast, levels of low-density lipoprotein increase with age in women. Levels of LDL are lower in females than males during youth and middle age but after menopause levels rise and are higher than men of similar age. A 1 mg/dl increase in HDL-C decreases CHD risk by 3% in women compared to 2% in men. Women have an average HDL-C of 55 mg/dl compared to 45 mg/dl in men.

Age at which twice the body mass at birth is reached is 3.6 months for boys and 4.1 months for girls. During exercise females oxidize proportionately more lipid and less carbohydrate, but the oxidation of amino acids is lower than in men. Females tend to have a blunted nighttime rise in PTH compared to men. Men have higher hepatic lipase levels than women. Hepatic lipase activity is 50% higher in males. The urinary excretion of cortisol and androgen metabolites is greater in males. Among older healthy adults, DHEA(S) levels are lower and cortisol levels higher in women. Homocysteine levels are higher in boys (5.22

umol/L) than in girls (4.84 umol/L). Calcitonin gene-related peptide-like immunoreactivity is higher in females. Normal women show greater glucose uptake per unit muscle mass than normal men after ingesting similar amount of glucose. The predominant tendency toward utilizing glucose by a nonoxidative pathway is more marked in normal women than in normal men for three hours after ingesting similar amount of glucose. Muscle insulin sensitivity appears to be greater in women.

Endocrine Laboratory Values

Androstenedione
 Female: 3.5–7.0 nmol/L
 Male: 3.0–5.0 nmol/L

Cortisol
 8 AM — Male: 16±1.7 nmol/L
     Female: 9.8±3.1 nmol/L
 8 PM — Male and Female: 3.9±0.2 nmol/L

Calcitonin Levels
 Male: 3–26 ng/liter
 Female: 2–17 ng/liter

Dehydroepiandrosterone (DHEA) Adult
 Male: 6.24–43.3 nmol/liter
 Female: 4.5–34.0 nmol/liter

Dehydroepiandrosterone Sulfate (Adult)
 Male: 100–6190 ug/liter
 Female:
  Premenopausal 120–5350 ug/liter
  Postmenopausal 300–2600 ug/liter

Dihydrotestosterone
 Female: 0.17–1 nmol/L
 Male: 0.87–2.6 nmol/L

Epinephrine
 Levels lower in women than men, but norepinephrine levels same

Estradiol
 Male: < 184 pmol/liter
 Female:
  Premenopausal

          Follicular phase   184–532 pmol/liter
          Midcycle peak   411–1626 pmol/liter
          Luteal phase   184–885 pmol/liter
          Postmenopausal   < 217 pmol/liter

Follicle Stimulating Hormone
    Male: 1.0–12.0 U/liter
    Female:
        Premenopausal
            Follicular phase   3.0–20.0 U/liter
            Ovulatory phase   9.0–26.0 U/liter
            Luteal phase   1.0–12.0 U/liter
        Postmenopausal   18.0–153.0 U/liter

17-Hydroxyprogesterone (Adult)
    Male: 0.15–7.5 nmol/liter
    Female:
        Premenopausal
            Follicular phase   0.6–3.0 nmol/liter
            Midcycle peak   3.0–7.5 nmol/liter
            Luteal phase   3.0–15.0 nmol/liter
        Postmenopausal   < 2.1 nmol/liter

Insulin-Like Growth Factor 1
    Male: 0.34–1.9 kU/L
    Female: 0.45–2.2 kU/L

17-Ketosteroids
    Male: 24.3–69.3 umol/24 hr
    Female: 17.3–52.0 umol/24 hr

Luteinizing Hormone
    Male: 2.0–12.0 U/liter
    Female:
        Premenopausal
            Follicular phase   2.0–15.0 U/liter
            Midcycle peak   22.0–105.0 U/liter
            Luteal phase   0.6–19.0 U/liter
        Postmenopausal   16.0–64.0 U/liter

Progesterone
    Male: < 3.18 nmol/liter

Female:
    Follicular phase   < 3.18 nmol/liter
    Midluteal phase   9.54–63.6 nmol/liter

Prolactin
    Male: 0–15 ug/liter
    Female:
        Premenopausal   0–20 ug/liter
        Postmenopausal   0–15 ug/liter

Sex Hormone Binding Globulin
    Male: 6–44 mmol/liter
    Female: 8–85 mmol/liter

Testosterone, Total (morning sample)
    Male: 9.36–37.1 nmol/liter
    Female: 0.21–2.98 nmol/liter

Testosterone, Unbound (morning sample)
    Female:
        20–40 yr   20.8–107.5 pmol/liter
        41–60 yr   13.9–86.7 pmol/liter
        61–80 yr   6.9–69.3 pmol/liter
    Male:
        20–40 yr   520–1387 pmol/liter
        41–60 yr   451–1213 pmol/liter
        61–80 yr   416–971 pmol/liter

Diseases

Addison's Disease
    Females > Males (2:1)

Adrenal Hypoplasia Congenita
    Male > Female
    Female carriers rarely have symptoms.

Adrenal Tumor
    Female > Male (3:1)

Aldosteronism, Idiopathic
    Male > Female

Aldosteronism, Primary
    Female > Male
    For adrenal adenoma

Amyloidosis
    Male > Female (2:1)

Autoimmune Adrenal Insufficiency
    With Polyglandular Autoimmune Syndrome
        Female > Male (7:3)
            Autoantibodies are more common in females.
    Isolated Autoimmune Adrenal Insufficiency
        Male > Female (7:3)
            In the first two decades of life.
        Female = Male
            In the 3rd decade.
        Female > Male (4:1)
            4th decade onwards.

Chorionic-Gonadotropin Secreting Tumor
    Male > Female
    Rare in females

Congenital Adrenal Hyperplasia
    Male = Female
    C4P21A2 *deficiency*
        Female infants virilized, but affected males have normal sexual development. Female are often infertile, while men may remain fertile.
    CYP17 *deficiency*
        Females have primary ammennorrhea and absent secondary sexual characteristics.
        Males usually have complete male pseudohermaphroditism with female external genitalia, a blind-ended vagina, and absence of uterus.
    3B-HSP *deficiency*
        Females have mild virilization of external genitalia.
        Males have varying degrees of failure of normal genital development ranging from hypospadias to male pseudohermaphroditism.

Congenital Hypothyroidism
   Female > Male (2–3:1)

Corticotrope Adenoma Subtype 1
   Female > Male

Corticotrope Adenoma Subtype 2
   Male > Female (4:1)

Corticotropin-Secreting Pituitary Adenoma
   Female > Male (8:1)

Cushing's Disease
   Female > Male (3–8:1)
   Females typically develop fine facial hair and males have decreased libido.

Cushing's Syndrome associated with Adrenal Tumor
   Female > Male (4–5:1)

Diabetes Insipidus
   Male > Female
   Usually X-linked recessive mode of inheritance. Expressed in males, rarely in females.

Diabetes Mellitus Type 1
   Male > Female (3:2)
         Of European origin
   There is ~ 2.5 year delay in onset of puberty in boys, the total pubertal height gain being normal. In girls, age of menarche is delayed and total pubertal height gain is diminished.
   Females are 1.5 times more likely to develop diabetic ketoacidosis; however the long term outcome is also better in females, as mortality is higher in males, especially black males.
   Females have higher values of plasma alpha 1-antitrysin than men. Fathers with type 1 DM are more likely than affected mothers to transmit the condition to their offspring.
   Autoantibodies are more frequent in female diabetes mellitus patients against both glutamic acid decarboxylase and tyrosine phosphatase.
   Compared to men, the inherent counterregulatory responses are decreased in healthy and Type 1 diabetic women. Men usually have an increased sympathetic nervous system counterregulatory response to hypoglycemia. Despite this, the prevalence of hypo-

glycemia is gender neutral. It appears that antecedent hypoglycemia produces less blunting of counterregulatory responses to subsequent hypoglycemia in women relative to men.

Males develop retinopathy more rapidly than females.

Amputations are 1.4–2.7 times higher in males.

Diabetes Mellitus Type 2

Female > Male (3.4:2.3)

HDL cholesterol is a protective factor in type 2 diabetes in women but not seen in men.

Shin spots occur in 1/2 of men and 1/3 of women over age 30 with diabetes mellitus Type 2.

Males with DM Type 2 appear to lose bone mass at a faster rate than nondiabetic males. This change is not seen in females.

Obesity is more common in women with DM Type 2 than in men with it.

Women with the disease have a poorer prognosis after MI than males with diabetes.

Women with the disease have increased risk of depression compared to male patients.

Increased risk of coronary artery disease 3–7 times in women versus 2–3 times in men.

Females have a higher prevalence of diagnosed diabetes, a greater reduction in life expectancy due to diabetes, and a higher incidence of ketoacidosis and hyperosmolar coma.

Women with DM have greater cardiovascular morbidity, and increased risks of new coronary events.

Women with DM have more significant coronary artery obstruction and multiple vessel disease, and a higher rate for restenosis than nondiabetic women. However men with DM have a higher prevalence of triple vessel disease but not stenosis compared to nondiabetic men.

Males with diabetes have twice the likelihood of death from heart disease compared to nondiabetic males. But diabetic women have five times the likelihood of death from heart disease as nondiabetic females.

Women are 4 times as likely and men 2 times as likely to develop heart failure as their nondiabetic counterparts.

Smoking and alcoholism appear to be more common in men with diabetes.

Females with DM are more likely to have increased LDL and triglycerides than men with DM.
Female with diabetes have a worse prognosis after stroke than males with DM.
Women with diabetes are more likely to suffer from blindness due to retinopathy than males with DM.
Neuropathy occurs more in women than in men with diabetes.
Men have more microalbuminuria and endstage renal disease than women with diabetes and are more likely to undergo kidney transplant.
Peripheral arterial disease is more common in men (21.3 vs. 17.6 per 1000 person years) than women with DM.
About 10% of women and 6% of men are blind because of diabetes.
Systolic blood pressure, regular smoking, and high daily alcohol intake are predictors of development of DM in men whereas uric acid and physical inactivity during leisure time are associated with the development of DM in women.
Women with the condition are more likely to transmit DM 2 to their offspring than men with the condition.

Diabetic Neuropathy
Sexual dysfunction seen in 30% of females and 50% of males.

Ectopic ACTH Syndrome
Male > Female (3:1)

Ectopic Corticotropin Syndrome
Male > Female

Familial Dysbetalipoproteinemia
Male > Female

Familial Hypercholesterolemia
Male = Female
But male heterozygotes die about 10 years earlier than female heterozygotes.

Familial Partial Lipodystrophy, Dunnigan Type
Males = Females
However women have a higher prevalence of diabetes (50% vs. 18%), and atherosclerotic heart disease (45% vs. 12%) and higher triglycerides (4.25 vs. 2.27 mmol/L) and lower HDL levels

(0.70 vs. 0.94 mmol/L). Women are more severely affected with metabolic complications of insulin resistance than men.

Galactorrhea
Female > Male (25:1)

Glucagonoma Syndrome
Female > Male

Glycoprotein-Producing Pituitary Adenoma
Male > Female

Gonadotrope Pituitary Adenoma
Male > Female
Gonadotropin level is usually increased in males but usually normal in females.

Graves' Disease
Female > Male (4–10:1)
In males, presents at a later age, is more severe, and accompanied more often by ophthalmopathy and myopathy.
In females, tends to become manifest in puberty, pregnancy, and at menopause.

Growth Hormone Deficiency
Male > Female
Males have greater response than females to the same dose of rhGH per body surface area with regard to changes in serum levels of IGF-1.

Hashimoto's Thyroiditis
Female > Male (25–50:1)

Hemochromatosis
Male = Female
But males are more likely (8:1) to show clinical signs.
Loss of blood in females (menstruation) delays onset of symptoms.
Usually diagnosed in males in their 5th decade; in women, 10–20 years after menopause.
Homozygous male relatives more likely to have a disease related condition than homozygous female relatives (38% vs. 10%).
Females are less likely to have cirrhosis of liver.
Of heterozygous carriers for hemochromatosis, 18% of males and 11% of females have transferrin saturation levels more than two

standard deviations above normal levels. Twenty percent of male heterozygotes and 8% of female heterozygotes have serum ferritin concentrations that exceed 95th percentile values.

Hypercholesterolemia
: Male > Female

Hypercholesterolemia, Familial
: Females = Male
: In heterozygotes, the average age of onset of coronary artery disease is 45 years in men, 55 years in women.
: In heterozygous familial hypercholestroemia, the cumulative probability of fatal or nonfatal coronary heart disease by age 60 years is 52% in men (versus 13% in men without) and 33% in women (versus 9% in women without familial hypercholesterolemia).

Hyperparathyroidism
: Female > Male (4:1)
: Prevalence in postmenopausal women may reach 3%.

Hyperprolactinemia
: Female > Male

Hyperthyroidism
: Female > Male (3:1)
: Affects 2% of women and 0.2% of men in their lifetime.
: 80% is due to Graves' disease.

Hypertriglyceridemia
: Male > Female

Hypoglycemia, Nondiabetic
: Female > Male

Hypokalemic Periodic Paralysis
: Male > Female (3:1)
:: Familial periodic paralysis onset is usually in late childhood or adolescence.
: Male > Female (13–20:1)
:: Hypokalemic periodic paralysis with thyrotoxicosis usually occurs in Asian males in early adulthood.

Hypothyroidism, Adult
: Female > Male (5–10:1)

Over age 65 years, 6–10% of women and 2–3% of men affected. Subclinical hypo and hyper thyroidism are more common in females.

Idiopathic Delayed Puberty
Male > Female

Idiopathic Diabetes Insipidus
Male > Female

Idiopathic Hypothyroidism
Female > Male

Idiopathic Sexual Precocity
Male > Female (10:1)
Precocious puberty is defined as androgen secretion and spermatogenesis before age 9–10 years in boys and onset of estrogen secretion and ovarian cycling in girls before age 8 years.

Insulinoma
Male > Female (3:2)

Kallman's Syndrome
Male > Female (4:1)

Lawrence-Seip Syndrome
Female > Male

Lesch-Nyhan Syndrome
Male > Female

Lithium-Induced Hypothyroidism
Female > Male

Lymphocytic Hypophysitis
Female > Male
Often occurs during pregnancy or postpartum.

McCune-Albright Syndrome
Female > Male (2:1)
Sexual precocity is seen in females, rarely in males.
Cafe' Au Lait spots and fibrous dysplasia are more common in females.

Nephrogenic Diabetes Insipidus
   Male > Female

Nonsecreting Pituitary Adenoma
   Occurs primarily in men and postmenopausal females.

Nontoxic Goiter
   Female > Male (7–9:1)
   More common during adolescence or pregnancy.

Osteoporosis
   Female > Male
   Lifetime risk for osteoporotic fracture in person over age 50 years is 40% in females and 13% in males.

   Lifetime risk of fracture in persons > 50 Years

	Female	Male
Proximal Femur	17.5%	6%
Vertebra	15.6%	5%
Distal Forearm	16%	2.5%
Average of the above	39.7%	13.1%

   Incidence of Collie's fracture increases in women as they age, but not in men.

Osteoporosis (Glucocorticoid-Induced)
   Female > Male

Overweight
   Females > Males
   In men the peak prevalence of overweight occurs between 45–54 years when it reaches a level of 31%, subsequently the prevalence of overweight decreases with age. In contrast, in women the prevalence of overweight increase throughout the entire age range reaching a peak of 38.5% in 65–74 year old women.
   8% of men and 10.8% of women are considered severe overweight. Morbid obesity (BMI of 39.0 or more in both sexes) occurs in 0.6% of males and 2.5% of females.
   Obesity is associated with an increase in postabsorptive plasma concentrations of branched-chain keto acids in men but not in women of similar BMI.
   In obese persons, men have larger internal fat cell sizes while women have larger subcutaneous fat cell sizes in the gluteal and femoral depots.

Paget's Disease
    Male ≥ Female
    Males are more symptomatic.

Pheochromocytoma
    Female > Male (slightly)

Polyglandular Autoimmune Syndrome I
    Female roughly equal to Male (0.8–1.7:1)
    Gonadal failure is more common in females than males (60% vs. 14%).

Polyglandular Autoimmune Syndrome II
    Female > Male (1.8:1)

Postoperative Hyponatremia
    Male = Female
    However females have a 25 times increased risk of death or permanent neurologic damage.

Precocious Puberty
    Female > Male (5:1)
    Idiopathic form 8 times more common in females
    Neurologic form is as common as the idiopathic form in males but only 1/5 as common as the idiopathic form in females.

Premature Adrenarche
    Females > Males
    In girls, increased risk for development of insulin resistance and ovarian hperandrogenism, especially polycystic ovary syndrome. It is usually a benign, self-limiting condition in boys.

Primary Adrenal Insufficiency
    Female > Male
    Females are more likely to have decreased axillary and pubic hair and loss of libido than males.
    Males may have calcification of auricular cartilage of the ear.
    Males have normal serum testosterone levels but females have low levels.

Primary Hyperparathyroidism
    Female > Male (2:1)

Primary Myxedema
:   Female > Male

Prolactinoma
:   Female > Male
    Up to 20% of females with unexplained amenorrhea have prolactinoma.
    Microadenoma is more common in females; macroadenoma is more common in males.
    Galactorrhea occurs in 30–80% of females and 14–33% of males.

Reidel's Thyroiditis
:   Female > Male

Subacute Thyroiditis
:   Female > Male

Suprasellar Germinoma
:   Male > Female

Thyroid Cancer
:   Female > Male (2.5–4:1)
        Papillary
    Female > Male (2:1)
        Poorly Differentiated (insular)
    Female > Male (1.3–1.5:1)
        Anaplastic
    Female > Male (slightly)
        Medullary

Thyroid Hormone Deficiency
:   Female > Male (10–20:1)

Thyroiditis
:   Female > Male
        Overall
    Female > Male
        Acute
    Female > Male (25:1)
        Chronic Lymphocytic
    Female > Male (3:1)
        Invasive Fibrous

> Female > Male (4:1)
>> Subacute Granulomatous

Thyroid Neoplasia, Malignant
> Female > Male (2.6:1)

Thyroid Nodule
> Female > Male (5–6:1)
> More likely to be malignant in males.

Thyrotoxic Periodic Paralysis
> Male > Female
> Primarily seen in Asian men.

Thyrotropin-Secreting Pituitary Adenoma
> Female > Male (1.7:1)

Toxic Multinodular Goiter
> Female > Male

Trimethylaminouria
> Females have more body odor than males with this condition.

Virilizing Adrenal Hyperplasia
> An affected female fetus is virilized with enlargement of the clitoris and fusion of the labia. These effects often lead to early detection and treatment. Unfortunately the male fetus does not usually show external features of the illness and may go undetected and present with salt wasting and shock.

Nephrology/Urology

Anatomy and Physiology

The kidneys of adult males weigh 230–440 (average 313) grams while for adult females 200–280 (average 250) grams.

Normal thickness of the glomerular basement membrane in adults:

Male: 373 ± 42 nm
Female: 326 ± 45 nm

Male urethra is 20 cm in length in adults. Female urethra is 5 cm in length in adults. The kidney increases 1 cm in length during pregnancy due to an increase in renal vascular volume and capacity of the collecting system as well as to hypertrophy of the kidney. The striated muscle of the external urethral sphincter surrounds the urethra circumferentially in males but in women the muscle separates posteriorly in the midline to accommodate the vagina. In men the bladder is better supported by the pelvic floor. Women have a posterior opening in the urogenital diaphragm that allows the bladder to descend, interfering with the urethrovesical junction which causes urethral insufficiency and allows bladder hypermobility. The peritoneal membrane is continuous and forms a closed space in males. In females, it is continuous with the membranes of the fallopian tubes. In the female, the wolffian duct and its associated mesonephric kidney undergoes dissolution. In the male, the wolffian duct becomes in part the vas deferens while the cranial complement of mesonephric tubules becomes the tubules of the epididymis. An epithelial evagination of the wolffian duct, the ureteric bud, sets the stages for development of the permanent kidneys in both sexes.

The total body water of young men is 60% of body weight and declines to 54% in men > 60 years. In young women, total body water is 51% of body weight and declines to 46% in females > 60 years.

The diastolic blood pressure increases until age 50 years in both males and females. The mean systolic pressure is lower in females under age 60 years. After age 60 years, it increases at a greater rate in females and is as high as corresponding values in males.

Young ovulating females excrete more kallikrein in their urine than either males or postmenopausal females. During the follicular period, the levels are similar to males. The rise occurs during the luteal phase of the cycle. The level of kallikrein excretion is diminished in essential hypertension. In adult males the serum phosphorous decreases from 3.5 mg/dl at age 20 years to 3.0 mg/dl at age 70 years. However postmenopausal females have a slightly higher serum phosphorous level of 3.7 mg/dl than premenopausal females of 3.4 mg/dl.

With advancing age and loss of muscle mass, the total body potassium and total exchangeable potassium levels decrease. This is more pronounced in females.

The urinary excretion of inositols is higher in males.

Renal Laboratory Values

Creatinine Excretion
  Varies by sex and age:
    In males 20–50 years old, the excretion is 25 mg/kg/day.
    In females 20–50 years old, the excretion is 16.5–22.4 mg/kg/day.
    In males 50–70 years, it decreases to 15.7–20.2 mg/kg/day.
    In females 50–70 yrs, it decreases to 11.8–16.1 mg/kg/day.

Serum Creatinine
  Men: 0.5–1.3 mg/dl
  Women: 0.5–1.1 mg/dl

To Estimate Creatinine Clearance
  For Male: $CrCl = \dfrac{(140 - age) \times (lean\ body\ weight)}{72 \times Serum\ creatinine}$
  For Female: CrCl = CrCl (calculated) x 0.85
  Lean body weight male = 50 + (2.3 x height in inches over 5 feet)
  Lean body weight female = 45.5 + (2.3 x height in inches over 5 feet)

Normal Urine Calcium Excretion
  Male: up to 300 mg/24 hours
  Female: up to 250 mg/24 hours

Upper limit of Daily Uric Acid Excretion
    Male: 800 mg
    Female: 750 mg

Angiotensin Converting Enzyme
    Male: 19–95 U/liter
    Female: 19–79 U/liter

Uric Acid
    Male: 214–506 umol/liter
    Female: 137–393 umol/liter

Mean Renal Plasma Flow
    Male: 655 ml/min/1.73 m^2
    Female: 600 ml/min/ 1.73 m^2

Glomerular Filtration Rate
    Male: 130 ml/min/1.73 m^2
    Female: 120 ml/min/1.73 m^2

Diseases

Acquired Renal Cystic Disease
    Male > Female
    Males are 4–7 times more likely to have neoplasms arising from the cystic lining compared to females.

Acute Glomerulonephritis
    Male > Female (3:2)
    Occurs mainly in children between 2–8 years of age.

Acute Poststreptococcal Glomerulonephritis
    Male > Female
    Male are more likely to have overt nephritis.

Acute Pyelonephritis
    Female > Male

Alport Syndrome
    Male > Female
    Males have persistent hematuria with episodes often exacerbated by infection or exercise.

Slowly progressive renal failure is common in males. Endstage renal disease often occurs in males between ages 16–35 years.

The disease is mild and only partially expressed in females. The prognosis in females is generally benign and most women survive into old age.

Analgesic Nephropathy
Female > Male (5–7:1)

Anti-Glomerular Basement Membrane Disease
Male > Female (1.1:1)
Two age peaks: the first is in the 2nd–3rd decade, has a male predominance, and higher frequency of lung hemorrhage. The second peak is in the 6th to 7th decade, has a female predominance, and more likely to have renal limited disease.

Atheroembolic Renal Disease
Male > Female (3–4:1)

Autosomal Dominant Polycystic kidney Disease
Female = Male
But male gender is a predisposing factor for renal disease progression.

Bladder Cancer
Male > Female (3:1)
4th most common cancer in males, 8th most common cancer in females.
Women that smoke have a higher risk of bladder cancer than men who smoke comparably.

Bladder Neck and Urethral Obstruction
Male > Female

Bladder Stones
Male > Female (9.5:1)

C-1q Nephropathy
Male > Female (1.8:1)

Calciphylaxis
Female > Male (6:1)
When it occurs in end-stage renal disease.

Collapsing Glomerulopathy in Focal Segmental Glomerulosclerosis
Male > Female (1.2:1)

Congenital Nephrogenic Diabetes Insipidus
Male > Female

Congenital Right Ureter Obstruction
Male > Female (3:1)
Due to abnormal development of venous system with obstruction from the inferior vena cava.

Congenital Uteropelvic Junction Obstruction
Male > Female (2:1)
60% occur on the left side.

Congenital Vesicoureteral Reflux
Male > Female (5:1)

Cystinuria
Female > Male
But males have more severe disease.

Cystitis
Female > Male

Dent Disease
Male > Female
Only males develop renal failure.

Diabetic Nephropathy
Male > Female
Microalbumiuria in both insulin dependent and noninsulin dependent diabetes mellitus is more common in males.

End-Stage Renal Disease
Male > Female
Rate of progression to ESRD is greater in males for various diseases such as hypertension, polycystic kidney disease and chronic glomerulonephritis.
The prevalence of hypertension is greater in men, men consume more protein, and dyslipidemia is greater in men than premenopausal females. All of these contribute to increased renal disease severity in males.

Enuresis
    Male > Female (2–3:1)
        Age 5 years: 7% of males, 3% of females
        Age 10 years: 3% of males, 2% of females
        Age 18 years: 1% males and even fewer females
        Noctural: Male > Female
        Daytime wetting: Female > Male

Essential Mixed Cryoglobulinemia
    Female > Male

Exstrophy of Bladder
    Male > Female (3–5:1)

Fabry Disease
    Male > Female
    Males have more severe disease. In males renal failure develops by the fifth decade.

Fibrillary Glomerulonephritis
    Female > Male (1.2–1.8:1)

Focal Glomerular Sclerosis (Collapsing)
    Male > Female

Focal Segmental Glomerular Sclerosis
    Male > Female (1.4:1)
        Typical
    Female > Male
        Tip Lesion

Glomerulonephritis, Acute
    Male > Female (3:2)

Glomerulonephritis, Poststreptococcal
    Male > Female (2:1)

Goodpasture's Syndrome
    Male > Female (6:1)

Hepatorenal Syndrome
    Male > Female

Heroin-Induced Nephropathy
    Male > Female (9:1)

Hydronephrosis
    Male = Female
        Age 0–20 years
    Female > Male
        Age 20–60 years
    Male > Female
        Age greater than 60 years
    Etiology of hydronephrosis
    Male > Female (65% male)
        Ureteropelvic junction obstruction
    Female > Male (7:1)
        Ureterovesicle junction obstruction secondary to ureterocele
    Male > Female
        Posterior urethral valves
    Male > Female (97% male)
        Prune belly syndrome

Hyperparathyroidism
    Female > Male

Hyponatremia
    Female > Male
    More severe in females at the same level of hypotonicity.

Hypophosphatemic Vitamin D-Resistant Rickets
    Male > Female (1.8:1)
        For bone disease

Idiopathic Edema
    Female > Male

Idiopathic Hypercalciuria
    Male > Female

IgA Nephropathy
    Male > Female (2–6:1)
    Male gender and older age at onset are poor prognostic factors.

Incontinence, Urinary
    Female > Male (5:1)
    Between 15–64 years of age, 1.5–5% of males and 10–25% of females affected.

Over age 50 years, up to 24% of males and 49% of females in one large study had incontinence. Men were more likely to seek treatment for incontinence (29% vs. 13%) in this study.

Blacks are 2 times as likely to have detrusor instability but one-half as likely to have stress incontinence as whites.

In females over age 65 years, 36% have experienced urge incontinence and 40% have experienced stress incontinence.

Interstitial Cystitis
    Female > Male (9–10:1)

Kidney Cancer
    Male > Female (3:2)

Kidney Cyst
    Female > Male

Kidney Stones
    Male > Female (4:1)
    Prevalence varies in men from 4–9% and in females from 1.7–4.1%.
        Males > Females
            Calcium oxalate
        Females > Males
            Struvite
        Females > Males
            Calcium phosphate
        Male = Female
            Cysteine Stones
        Male > Female
            Uric Acid Stones

Lipodystrophy
    Female > Male
    Primary lipodystrophy often presents in girls between ages 5–15 years and renal disease occurs in 20–50% of these cases.

Loin Pain Hematuric Syndrome
    Female > Male
    Primarily in young women, oral contraceptives have been associated with this condition.

Lowe Syndrome
    Male > Female
    Renal, ocular and neurologic defects are seen.

Malacoplakia
    Female > Male (4:1)

Medullary Sponge Kidney
    Male = Female
    But infections are more common in females.
    Hypercalciuria found in 45% of males and 26% of females.
    Females with nephrolithiasis are twice as likely to develop medullary sponge kidney.

Membranoproliferative Glomerulonephritis: Type I
    Male > Female (1.2:1)

Membranous Glomerulopathy
    Male > Female (2:1)
    Most common cause of nephrotic syndrome in adults.
    Males are more likely to progress to chronic renal failure.

Membranous Nephropathy
    Male > Female (2:1)
        Nonlupus related; males have more severe disease.
    Female > Male
        Lupus related

Mesangial Proliferative Glomerulonephritis
    Male > Female

Minimal Change Glomerulopathy
    Male > Female (1.1:1)
        Adult
    Male > Female (2–2.5:1)
        In children

Nephrogenic Diabetes Insipidus (Familial)
    Male > Female

Nephrotic Syndrome
    Male > Female (3:2)
        Overall

Male > Female
: In young children

Male = Female
: In adolescents

Orthostatic Proteinuria
: Male > Female

Perinatal Acidemia — Severe
: Male > Female

Periurethral Abscess
: Male > Female

Polycystic Kidney Disease, Autosomal Dominant
: Male = Female
: But worse prognosis in males.

Posterior Urethral Valves
: Male > Female

Primary Amyloidosis
: Male > Female (2:1)

Primary Hypomagnesemia
: Male > Female (3:1)
: Due to inherited defect in intestinal magnesium absorption.

Pyelonephritis
: Female > Male
: Predominant age — Sexually active years in women, but > 50 years in men.

Renal Artery Aneurysm
: Female > Male
  : Fusiform variety
  : Pregnancy is a risk factor for renal artery aneurysm rupture.
: Male > Female
  : Saccular variety
: Male > Female (3:1)
  : Dissecting variety
  : Occurs primarily on the right side.

Renal Artery Stenosis
: Male > Female

Nephrology/Urology

Atherosclerotic
Female > Male
Fibromuscular dysplasia and Takayasu's arteritis

Renal Calculi
Male > Female (3–4:1)
Except struvite stones which are more common in females.

Renal Cell Adenocarcinoma
Male > Female (9.6:4.2)
9th most common male malignant tumor, 13th most common female malignant tumor, but the gender gap is closing. Rate increased from 0.7 to 4.2 per 100,000 from 1935 to 1989 in females. Rate increase from 1.6 to 9.6 per 100,000 for males in this same time period.

Renal Pelvis Carcinoma
Male > Female (2:1)

Renal Transplant
Overall graft survival and patient survival appear better in female recipients.
Females have greater risk of acute rejection but lower risk of chronic allograft failure than men.
Factors that negatively influence graft survival:
Male recipient, especially from female donor.
Small kidneys from women, small children or black donors fail sooner than large kidneys from white donors.

Renal Vascular Hypertension
Female > Male
< 50 years
Usually due to fibromuscular dysplasia
Male > Female
> 50 years
Usually due to atherosclerosis

Renal Vein Thrombosis
Male > Female (slightly)

Rhabdomyolysis
Male > Female
Due to more overall trauma in males.

Sarcoidosis with Granulomatous Interstitial Nephritis
    Male > Female

Schonlein-Henoch Purpura
    Male > Female (2:1)

Scleroderma
    Female > Male (3:1)
    Ratio increases to 15:1 during the childbearing years.
    Renal involvement includes chronic renal disease or scleroderma renal crisis.

Solitary Multilocular Cysts
    38% of lesions in males occur in the first 3 years of life, whereas in females, 37% of lesions present between ages 1–15 years and 63% present between ages 31–69 years.

Systemic Lupus Erythematosus
    Female > Male
    However males with SLE have same incidence of renal disease as females.

Thrombotic Thrombocytopenic Purpura
    Female > Male (3–5:2)
    Renal involvement in 80–90%.
    Male sex associated with greater risk of renal sequelae.

Transitional Cell Cancer of Kidneys and Ureters
    Female > Male

Urate Nephropathy
    Male > Female

Ureteral Obstruction
    Female > Male

Ureteral Tumor
    Male > Female (3:1)

Ureteropelvic Junction Obstruction
    Male > Female (2–4:1)

Urethral Cancer
    Male > Female (3:1)

Urethral Diverticula
    Female > Male

Urethral Injury
    Male > Female
    Due to the male urethra attachment to the pubis by the puboprostatic ligament and the suspensory ligament of the penis.

Urethral Prolapse
    Female > Male

Urethral Valve Narrowing
    Male > Female

Urethritis
    Male = Female
    But classic symptoms more common in males.
    Gonorrhea is a common cause in men but rarely in women.

Urinary Incontinence
    Female > Male (8:1)
    In a study of people over age 50 years, 24% of males and 49% of females reported incontinence. Of these, 29% of men but only 13% of women sought medical treatment.
    An estimated 13 million adults suffer from incontinence; 11 million of these are females.
    Stress incontinence is common in females but unusual in males and usually the result of urologic surgery in males.
    Males are more likely to have urge incontinence.
    Men are less susceptible to stress incontinence due to longer urethra through which more pressure is needed to move urine. The angulation of the male urethra may contribute to urethral resistance also.
    Mixed incontinence is more common in females.
    Males suffer incontinence primarily due to bladder outlet obstruction.
    Urinary dysfunction in men is usually due to disorders of the bladder emptying phase. Disorders of urine storage in men occur usually in the setting of severe neurological disease and its associated detrusor hyperreflexia, or more commonly after radical prostate surgery.
    In women, bladder dysfunction is usually due to deficits of urine storage. Urge, stress and mixed incontinence are the primary con-

ditions in women. Disorders of bladder emptying are less common in women and are often due to severe prolapse, prior vaginal surgery, paraurethral masses or neurological disorders.

Stress incontinence in men is usually due to prostatectomy-related scarring of the bladder neck.

Urinary Tract Infection
- Female > Male (14:1)
  - Adults
  - Uncommon in men < 50 years.
  - In adults > 65 years, 10% of men and 20% of females have bacteriuria.
  - Males are more likely to have lower urinary tract obstruction.
  - Females are more likely to have neurogenic bladder, infected stones, vesicoureteral reflux and hydronephrosis.
- Female > Male (>30:1)
  - Young adults
  - 1–3% of females between 15–24 years have bacteriuria increasing to 10–15% by the 6th to 7th decade of life.
  - Dysuria occurs each year in 20% of females between 24–64 years, two-thirds of who have significant bacteriuria with clinical symptoms.
  - Bacteriuria occurs in 4–10% of pregnant women.
  - Bacteriuria is unusual in males before age 50 years occurring in only 0.04–0.14%.
- Male > Female (2–4:1)
  - Neonates
  - Due to structural abnormalities.
  - Uncircumsized males are at increased risk of infection.
  - Asymptomatic bacteriuria is more common in male infants.
- Female > Male (9–15:1)
  - Preschool children
  - 8% of females and 2% of males will have a UTI in childhood.
  - 20% of schoolgirls with UTI have vesiculoureteral reflux.
  - The frequency of neurologic and structural defects in boys with UTI is higher than in girls with UTI.
  - 1% of preschool girls and fewer boys have asymptomatic bacteriuria.

Male > Female
> Elderly
>> Age > 55 years, is primarily due to due to prostate disease in men.
>> By age 70 years, 3.5% of males have bacteriuria and the frequency increases with debilitation.

Urinary Tract Obstruction
> Female > Male
>> Age 20–60 years, primarily due to pregnancy and uterine cancer in women.
> Male > Female
>> Age > 60 years, primarily due to prostate disease in men. End stage renal disease due to obstruction is more common in males.

Urolithiasis
> Male > Female (4:1)
>> Overall
> Male > Female (1.5:1)
>> After sixth decade

Vesiculoureteral Reflux
> Female > Male (5:1)
>> Early childhood
> Male > Female
>> Infancy

Wilms' Tumor
> Female > Male (1.1:1)
> Especially for bilateral disease.

Xanthogranulomatous Pyelonephritis
> Female > Male (2:1)

X-linked Hypophosphatemic Rickets
> Male > Female
> Males more severely affected.

X-linked Nephrogenic Diabetes Insipidus
> Male > Female
> Mental retardation occurs in males.

Allergy/Immunology

Anatomy and Physiology

Females have better B-cell mediated immunity than age-matched males. Females have higher immunoglobulin levels, stronger antibody responses to foreign antigens, and increased resistance to some infections. Females have greater resistance to induced tolerance, increased ability to reject grafts, and increased CD4 to CD8 ratios, secrete higher levels of interleukin-4 and interleukin-1 and gamma-interferon than males. Serum IgE levels: Children (males and females) have similar levels, but adult males have significantly higher levels than adult females. The male immune system does not have the degree of sensitivity as the female system. Women have an immune system that is geared to maintain a fetus for 9 months, and is sensitive to any shift in hormone levels, change in diet, or environmental influences. This is why many fertility problems occur in females with autoimmune disease. The male immune system is less complex and is geared to reject foreign invaders such as bacterial pathogens.

Men are found to have higher levels of IL-2 and lower levels of IL-4 and IL-10 than women. IgE levels increase in both sexes of children but boys have higher levels than girls by age 2–4 years. This may partially explain the higher frequency of allergic disease, especially asthma, in boys. Immunoglobulin levels vary between the sexes and levels of certain ones such as IgG and IgM are higher in females than in males in response to antigenic challenge. CD4 lymphocye levels are also higher in women. Females have higher levels of immunoglobulins, greater antibody response to antigens and more autoimmune diseases. Females appear to have better thymic function than men. Females have a higher number of recent thymic emigrants for longer periods of life in their peripheral blood than men. Evidence of sex steroids effect on certain autoimmune diseases is noted by improvement of symptoms in rheumatoid arthritis patients, but not lupus patients, during pregnancy.

In males, the absence of testosterone results in the synthesis of certain autoantibodies. In many women the autoantibodies already exist and the ingestion of agents such as exogenous estrogen can enhance the titer of these antibodies even in the absence of disease. No one with antiphospholipid syndrome should ingest estrogenic hormones as this may increase likelihood of blood clots forming.

Cell mediated immune processes are depressed in men after traumatic hemorrhage whereas they are unchanged or increased in females. It appears that androgens are responsible for the immunodepression after trauma. In contrast, females' sex steroids appear to have immunoprotective properties after trauma.

Globally, estrogens depress T-cell dependent immune functions and diseases, but enhance antibody production and aggravate B-cell dependent diseases. Androgens suppress both B-cell and T-cell immune responses and usually result in the suppression of disease expression. The glucocorticoid response to stress, including immune challenge, is enhanced by estrogens and inhibited by androgens.

Skin Testing: There is no difference between men and women for allergy testing. However, women exhibit weakest histamine capacity at the day of the menstrual cycle and a second minimum around the 20th day of the cycle. In some studies, females are less responsive to the antigens in the Multitest CMI skin test preparation for delayed-type hypersensitivity than are men.

Diseases

Acute Eosinophilic Pneumonia
    Male > Female

Acute Otitis Media
    Male > Female

Allergic Rhinitis
    Male > Female (slightly)
    In people 12 to 74 years old, 6.3% of males and 8.7% of females report AR.
    In children, boys are 2 times more affected than girls.
    Males are two times more likely to remit.

Anaphylactic Reaction
    Female = Male
        In general
    Females > Males
        For intravenous muscle relaxants, latex, aspirin
    Male > Female
        Insect stings

Asthma
    Male > Female
        Children
    Boys have smaller airways for a given lung size than girls. Also lower air flow rates occur in boys 4–6 years of age in addition to higher airways resistance compared to girls of the same age.
    Gender does not appear to affect the course of the disease.
    Risk of developing asthma in boys <10 years is about 2 times greater than in girls, and by the age of 14 years, boys are 4 times more likely to have chronic asthma and are 2 times more likely to be hospitalized. During and after adolescence however, post-pubertal females are at slightly greater risk of developing asthma and three times more likely to be hospitalized.

Chronic Eosinophilic Pneumonia
    Female > Male (2:1)

Chronic Granulomatous Disease
    Male > Female
    65% of cases are X-linked.

Churg Strauss Syndrome
    Male > Female (2:1)

Food Allergy
    Male > Female (2:1)

Histiocytosis Syndrome
    Male > Female (2:1)
        Class 1
    Male = Female
        Class II

Hypereosinophilic Syndrome
    Male > Female (9:1)

154 Allergy/Immunology

Immunodeficiency Diseases
　　Male > Female

Job Syndrome (Hyperimmunoglobulimemia E with Impaired Chemotaxis)
　　Female > Male

Langerhans Cell Histiocytosis
　　Male > Female (2:1)

Latex Sensitization
　　Male > Female (2:1)

Listeriosis
　　Pregnant women are more susceptible accounting for 1/3rd of reported cases.

Lower Respiratory Infections
　　Male > Female

Mastocytosis
　　Male > Female (1.5:1)

Mastocytosis, Indolent
　　Male sex is associated with worse prognosis.

Nasal Polyps
　　Male > Female (2:1)
　　Females with nasal polyps are two times more likely to have asthma.

Otitis Media with Middle Ear Diffusion
　　Male > Female

Primary Immunodeficiency
　　Male > Female (5:1)
　　　　Childhood, predominantly males are affected.
　　Female > Male (1.4:1)
　　　　Adult

Properiden Deficiency
　　Male > Female
　　Increases susceptibility to meningococcal infections.

Recurrent Otitis Media
　　Male > Female

Severe Combined Immunodeficiency Disease, X-linked
    Male > Female

Wiskott-Aldrich Syndrome
    Male > Female
    Rare in females, some carriers may express disease.

X-linked Agammoglobulinemia
    Male > Female
    Recurrent infections with encapsulated microbes are noted.

X-linked Hypogammaglobulinemia with Growth Hormone Deficiency
    Male > Female
    One half to one third of boys will develop rheumatoid-like arthritis.

X-linked Immunodeficiency with Hyper IgM
    Male > Female

X-linked Lymphoproliferative Disease
    Male > Female
    Infections with Epstein Barr virus, usually resulting in fatal malignancy, may occur.

X-linked Severe Combined Immunodeficiency
    Male > Female

Hematology/Oncology

Anatomy and Physiology

Sex chromatin (Barr) bodies are present in 80–90% of the somatic cells of normal females. It takes the form of a drumstick projection from the nuclear lobes of about 2–3% of segmented neutrophils in the blood of females. Eosinophils and probably basophils also have drumstick projections in females.

Testosterone induces apoptosis. Estrogen affects the coagulation profile. Fibrinogen levels and fibrinolytic activity are higher in females. Antithrombin III levels decline in men over age 40 years but not in women. Females have lower Protein S levels than males. Protein S is decreased during pregnancy and in females taking oral contraceptives. The urinary erythropoietin levels are 3 times higher in normal men than in normal women.

Polymorphisms of the erythropoietin gene or its receptor occur. The EPORA1 and EPORA10 alleles are more frequent in females and the EPOR5 allele is more common in males.

Platelet phenolsulfotransferase levels have different seasonal activities in the sexes. Platelet alpha 2-adrenergic receptor responsiveness is increased in elderly men but not elderly women. The concentration of 1,25 Dihydroxyvitamin D3 receptors in peripheral blood mononuclear cells is lower in females than males. Euglobulin clot lysis time is shorter in females. Tissue plasminogen activator and plasminogen activator inhibitor 1 are lower in females. The phase of the circadian rhythm of the fibrinolytic parameters may be advanced in females compared to males.

Serum TxB2 and cholesterol platelet membrane levels are higher in males than in females. In males, the platelet proaggregatory capacity is greater than in females. Peripheral blood mononuclear cells from females express a seven-fold higher vasopressin receptor density than in males.

Hematology Laboratory Values:

Normal values for Red Blood Cell, Plasma and Total Blood Volume— (ml/kg ± 1 std dev)

	RBC	Plasma	Total Blood Volume
Women	25.4 ± 2.6	36.8 ± 3.7	
	24.4 ± 2.6	34.8 ± 3.2	58.9 ± 4.9
Men	28.3 ± 2.8	34.4 ± 4.0	
	28.3 ± 4.1	33.5 ± 5.2	61.5 ± 8.6

Hemoglobin

Adults	Conventional Units	Range SI Units
Male:	14–17.4 g/dl	8.1–11.2 mmol/liter
	(lower limit of normal 13.2 g/dl)	
Female:	12.3–15.3 g/dl	7.4–9.9 mmol/liter
	(lower limit of normal 11.7 g/dl)	

The normal hemoglobin value for men decreases after age 65 years, but not in women.

Hematocrit   SI Units
    Male: 0.37–0.49
    Female: 0.36–0.46

Mean Corpuscular Volume
    Male: 78–100 fl
    Female: 78–102 fl

Serum Ferritin
    Adult men: 90–95 ug/L
    Adult women: 35 ug/L

During adolescence, the higher adult values of serum ferritin are established in young men. After menopause, values increase in women and approach levels of men. Serum ferritin values in men tend to rise steadily with age.

Erythrocyte Zinc Protoporphyrin—Hematoflorometric method
    Normal male (adult):   11 ug/dl   range 1–27
    Normal female (adult):   28 ug/dl   range 11–45

Iron deficient male: 103 ug/dl range 20–227
Iron deficient female: 73 ug/dl range 14–186

Iron Status of Normals, Heterozygotes and Homozgotes for Hemochromatosis

Normal	Male	Female
Serum iron (ug/dl)	106	96
Transferrin saturation (%)	31	29
Serrum ferritin (ng/ml)	135	72
Hepatic iron stain (grade 0–4)	0.3	0.1
Hepatic iron (ug/100 mg wet wt.)	12	7.9

Heterozygote	Male	Female
Serum iron	127	108
Transferrin saturation	42	35
Serum ferritin	155	64
Hepatic iron stain	1.1	1
Hepatic iron	105	72

Homozygote	Male	Female
Serum Iron	252	176
Transferrin saturation	95	74
Serum ferritin	1898	537
Hepatic iron stain	3.9	2.9
Hepatic iron	820	361

Frequency of Autoantibodies (%) to:

	Parietal Cells	Intrinsic Factor	Thyroid Cytoplasm
Men			
< 55 years	5.6%	very rare	5.2%
> 55 years	9.2%	<1%	
Women			
< 55 years	14.7%	very rare	12.2%
> 55 years	22.3%	<1%	

Prostate Specific Antigen
  Female: < 0.5 ug/liter
  Male:
    <40 years 0.0–2.0 ug/liter
    > 40 years 0.0–4.0 ug/liter

Leukocyte Alkaline Phosphatase Scores

	Mean	95% limits
Male:	73	22–124
Female:	91	33–149

Diseases

Acute Lymphocytic Leukemia
    Male > Female
    57% of cases occur in males.
    Male sex is associated with an unfavorable prognosis.
    T-cell acute lymphocytic leukemia is more common in males.
    Males are more likely to relapse after chemotherapy.

Acute Myelogenous Leukemia
    Male > Female (3:2)

Adult T-cell Leukemia
    Male > Female (1.3–2.2:1)

Agnogenic Myeloid Metaplasia
    Female = Male
        Adults
    Male > Female (2:1)
        Children

Alloantibodies Reacting with Leukocyte Antigens
    Female > Male
    Occurs primarily in multiparous females.

Anemia
    Female > Male
    Occurs in 3% of adult men and 4–6% of adult females.
    In females, iron deficiency occurs mostly during the reproductive years.
    In males, incidence higher during adolescence, then decrease during young adulthood, then increases with advanced age.

Antiphospholipid Syndrome
    Female > Male (5–9:1)

Autoerythrocyte Sensitization (Psychogenic Purpura)
    Female > Male

Autoimmune Hemolytic Anemia
    Female > Male (2:1)
    With ageing and the menopause, women with autoimmune disorders tend to improve and show less clinical disease activity as estrogen levels drop. In men, the prevalence of autoimmune disease increases with age as androgens decrease and estrogen remains unopposed.
    Young males whose testes have been removed are at increased risk for autoimmune disease.

Barth Syndrome
    Male > Female

Brain Cancer
    Male > Female (1.4:1)
    Overall

Breast Cancer
    Female > Male (99:1)
    Affected males tend to be older, have subareolar tumors and present in more advanced stages.
    Overall survival rates in males are lower.

Burkitt's Lymphoma
    Male > Female (2–3:1)

Cancer
    Male > Female (overall)
    Probability of developing cancer from all sites from birth to death is 43.5% in males and 38.1% in females.
    Females who are long term survivors of a first malignancy have a higher risk of a second cancer compared to men (19–49% vs. 2–19%)

    10 Leading Sites of New Cancer Cases by Gender, US 2000
    (excludes basal and squamous cell skin cancer)

Male	*Female*
Prostate 29%	Breast 30%
Lung/Bronchus 14%	Lung/Bronchus 12%
Colon/Rectum 10%	Colon/Rectum 11%

Urinary Bladder 6%	Uterus 6%
Non-Hodgkins 5%	Ovary 4%
Melanoma 4%	Non-Hodgkins Lympoma 4%
Oral/Pharynx 3%	Melanoma 3%
Kidney/Renal 3%	Urinary Bladder 2%
Leukemia 3%	Pancreas 2%
Pancreas 2%	Thyroid 2%
All Other Sites 19%	All Other sites 22%

10 Leading Sites by Gender for Cancer Deaths, US 2000

Male	*Female*
Lung/Bronchus 31%	Lung/Bronchus 25%
Prostate 11%	Breast 15%
Colon/Rectum 10%	Colon/Rectum 11%
Pancreas 5%	Pancreas 5%
Non-Hodgkins 5%	Ovary 5%
Leukemia 4%	Non-Hodgkins Lymphoma 5%
Esophagus 3%	Leukemia 4%
Liver/Bile 3%	Uterus 2%
Bladder 3%	Brain/nervous System 2%
Stomach 3%	Stomach 2%
	Multiple Myeloma 2%
All Other Sites 22%	All Other Sites 21%

Cerebral Meningioma
 Female > Male (1.5:1)

Chediak-Steinbrick-Higashi Anomaly
 Female > Male (10:8.7)

Chlorosis
 Female > Male
 Primarily in girls 14–17 years old.

Chronic Acquired Erythrocytic Hypoplasia
 Female > Male (3.5–4:1)
  With Thymoma
 Male > Female (2:1)
  Without Thymoma

Chronic Congenital Hemolytic Disease
 Females have more cholelithiasis than males.
 Leg ulcers are more common in males.

Chronic Granulomatous Disease
> Male > Female
> 2/3 are X-linked, 1/3 are autosomal recessive.

Chronic Idiopathic Thrombocytopenia
> Female > Male (3:1)

Chronic Lymphocytic Leukemia
> Male > Female (2:1)

Chronic Myeloid Leukemia
> Male > Female (3:2)

Cold Agglutinin Disease
> Female > Male

Congenital Erythroid Hypoplasia of Diamond-Blackfan
> Males are less clinically affected but the reason is unknown.

Congenital Folate Malabsorption
> Female > Male

Cutaneous T-Cell Lymphoma
> Male > Female (2:1)

Cyclic Thrombocytopenia
> Cycles usually do not correlate with menstrual cycle.
> Periodic increased destruction of platelets is more common in females.
> Periodic decreased production of platelets is more common in males.

Disorders of Coagulation
> Male > Female
> 80–90% of inherited disorders occur in males.

Disorders of Platelets or Vessels
> Relatively more common in females.

Dyskeratosis Congenita
> Male > Female

Erythrocytosis
> When males have a hematocrit > 60% or > 55% in females, then the probability is about 99% that the RBC mass is elevated.

Erythroleukemia
    Male > Female

Essential Thrombocythemia
    Female > Male

Fabry Disease
    Male > Female
    Males with Type B or AB blood groups have more severe disease.

Factor IX Deficiency
    Males only
    Affects 1 in 30,000

G6PD Deficiency
    Males > Females
    Males more severely affected.

Gaisbock Syndrome (Chronic Relative Polycythemia)
    Male > Female
    Obesity, smoking and hypertension are often associated.

Gamma Heavy Chain Disease
    Male > Female (slightly)

Germ Cell Tumor
    Girls—Peak age 10–14 years
    Boys—Peak age 0–4 years

Gilbert's Disease
    Male > Female (2–7:1)

Glioblastoma
    Male > Female (1.6:1)

Gliomas
    Male > Female (1.5:1)
    59% of primary brain cancer in males
    42% of primary brain cancer in females

Gonadotroph Adenoma
    The tumors in females are more well-differentiated, with a highly distinctive vesicular dilitation of the golgi complex. Males have poorly or moderately developed cytoplasmic organelles.

Hairy Cell Leukemia
  Male > Female (4:1)

Heckathorn's Disease
  Male > Female

Hemochromatosis
  Male = Female
  Clinical disease is more apparent in males.
  Females with the disease possess 40% as much mobilizable iron as men.
  Menstrual blood loss may explain why females develop less clinical disease.
  Males may experience loss of libido, impotence, loss of axillae hair.
  Females may experience premature menopause.
  Iron loaded individuals are susceptible to *Vibrio vulnificus* and *Yersinia enterocolitica* infections.

Hemolytic Transfusion Reactions
  Female > Male
  Usually because of prior red cell immunization during pregnancy.

Hemophagocytic Syndrome
  Male > Female (2:1)

Hemophilia A & B
  Male > Female
  Females are usually asymptomatic carriers.
  Hemophilia A: 100 cases per 1 million males
  Hemophilia B: 20 cases per 1 million males

Hepatosplenic T-Cell Lymphoma
  Male > Female

Histiocytic Disorder
  Male > Female (2:1)

Hodgkin's Disease
  Male > Female (1.4:1)
    Overall
  Male > Female (3–4:1)
    Children < 10 years
  Male > Female (1–3:1)

Older Children
In childhood Hodgkin's disease, 80% occurs in males

Hypereosinophilic Syndrome
Male > Female (9:1)

Hypergammaglobulinemic Purpura
Female > Male

Hypoferremia
Female > Male
In the US, 8.3% of men and 14% of women have decreased iron.

Hypogonadism
In eunuchoid or castrated males, the RBC concentration and blood hemoglobin concentration are within values of normal females. (Normally after puberty, values for VPRBC, Hemoglobin concentration and RBC count are 10–13% higher in men).

Hypothyroidism
Anemia in hypothyroidism is more common in males, although hypothyroidism is more common in females.

Idiopathic Hypereosinophilic Syndrome
Male > Female (9:1)

Idiopathic Thrombocytopenic Purpura
Male = Female
    Acute, usually seen in childhood
Female > Male (3–7:1)
    Chronic, usually seen in adults
    70% of affected females are under age 40 years.

Infection Associated Hemophagocytic Syndrome
Male > Female

Iron Deficiency Anemia
Female > Male
Incidence is equal in infants.
Adult men require 5–10 mg/day of iron, whereas adult women require 7–20 mg/day.
Menstrual blood loss is most common cause in women.
The normal menstrual period averages 35 ml with upper limit of normal of 80 ml blood loss per period.

Iron deficiency occurs in 5–30% of women and 1–4% of men, and is reported to be even more common in pregnant women and adolescents of both sexes.

Kamura's Disease
  Male > Female
  Primarily Asian males affected.

Kaposi's Sarcoma
  Male > Female

Langerhans Cell Histiocytosis
  Male > Female (slightly)
  In one series of patients with localized bone disease the male to female ratio was 1.8:1.

Leukemia
  Male > Female (13.2:7.7)

Leukemia, Acute Lymphoblastic in Adults
  Male > Female (slightly)

Leukemia, Chronic Lymphocytic
  Male > Female (2:1)

Leukemia, Hairy Cell
  Male > Female (4:1)
  Predominantly in men between 40 to 60 years of age.

Lymphedema
  Female > Male (3.5:1)

Lymphoblastic Leukemia
  Male > Female

Lymphoma
  Male > Female
  More men than women with stage B-type lymphatic lymphoma test positive for the MDR1 (multidrug resistant) phenotype. This may explain why women have a more benign course of disease.

Lymphoma Associated with Immunodeficiency States
  Male > Female
  In part because of the contribution of X-linked disorders.

Lymphoma Associated with Sjogren's Syndrome and Hashimoto's Thyroiditis
    Female > Male

Malignant Histiocytosis
    Male > Female

Mantle Cell Lymphoma
    Male > Female (4:1)

March Hemoglobinuria
    Male > Female
    Primarily appears in young men during prolonged exercise.

McCleod Phenotype of Heriditary Spherocytosis
    Male > Female

Medullary Plasmocytoma
    Male > Female

Medulloblastomas
    Male > Female
    In children

Meningioma
    Female > Male (9:5)
    20% of primary brain cancer in males.
    36% of primary brain cancer in females.

Multiple Myeloma
    Male > Female (4.7:3.3)

Myelodysplasia
    Male > Female (3:2)
    Male predominance seen in de novo and treatment related myelodysplasia. This may reflect sexual disparity in environmental exposures or the hematopoietic stimulatory effects of androgens.
    5 q-Syndrome: Females make up 70% of cases.

Myeloproliferative Disorders
    Male > Female (1.7:1)
        Chronic Myelogenous Leukemia
    Male > Female (slightly)
        Agnogenic myeloid metaplasia with myelofibrosis
    Female > Male (1.3:1)
        Essential Thrombocytosis

Neuroectodermal Tumor
    Male > Female (2:1)
        In children

Non-Hodgkin's Lymphoma
    Male > Female (2–3:1)
    Incidence is increasing, especially in elderly white males.

Osteosarcoma
    Female > Male
        (10–14 years)
    Male > Female
        (≥ 15 years)

Osteosclerotic Myeloma
    Male > Female

Paroxysmal Nocturnal Hemoglobinuria
    Female > Male (slightly)
    Pregnancy is often hazardous in females with this disorder.

Pernicious Anemia
    Female ≥ Male
    Prevalence highest in females (2.7%), especially in black females (4.3%).
    In US, distribution between sexes is equal, but in many countries, females predominate.
    About 30% of female relatives and 18% of male relatives of pernicious anemia patients have autoantibodies to parietal cells.

Pheochromocytoma
    Female = Male
    But female 3 times as likely to have malignant tumor.

Phosphoglycerate Kinase Deficiency
    Male > Female

Pica
    Female > Male

Polycythemia Vera
    Male > Female (1.2–2.2:1)

Porphyria
    Male > Female

Porphyria Cutanea Tarda
  Female > Male
Acute Intermittent Porphyria
  Female > Male
Variegate Porphyria
  Female > Male
Hereditary Coproporphyria
  Female > Male
Porphobilinogen Synthetase Deficiency

Primary Heriditary Sideroblastic Anemia
  Male > Female

Primary Mediastinal Large B-Cell Lymphoma
  Female > Male (2:1)

Primary Warm Autoimmune Hemolytic Disease
  Female > Male (2:1)

Reduced RBC Folate Levels
  Female > Male
  In North America, 8% of males and 12–13% of females have decreased folate levels but megaloblastic anemia is uncommon.

Rhabdosarcoma
  Male > Female (1.2–1.5:1)

Sickle Cell Anemia
  Male = Female
  However leg ulcers more common in males.
  Alloimmunization after transfusion is more common in females.

Sideroblastic Anemia, X-linked
  Male > Female

Spinal Meningioma
  Female > Male (3.5:1)

Superior Vena Cava Syndrome
  Male > Female

Teratoma
  Female > Male
  Excluding testicular teratomas, 80% occur in females.

Sacrococcygeal tumors are 4 times more common in females.
Teratomas account for 50% of all ovarian neoplasms.

Thrombotic Thrombocytopenic Purpura
Female > Male (2:1)
Primarily occurs between 10–50 years of age.

Transfusion Reaction, Hemolytic
Female > Male

Transient Erythroblastopenia of Childhood
Male > Female (1.4:1)

Waldenstrom's Macroglobulinemia
Male > Female (2–3:1)
Male gender associated with shorter survival.

Wilms' Tumor
Female > Male (slightly)

Wiskott-Aldrich Syndrome
Male > Female

X-linked Lymphoproliferative Disease
Male > Female
Patients usually have severe Epstein-Barr viral infections.

Gastroenterology

Anatomy and Physiology

Differences in the esophagus between the sexes include:

- slightly shorter length in females when matched for height;
- duration and velocity of contractions (women with and without reflux have higher amplitude of contractions than men with and without reflux);
- women have less physiological reflux;
- pain threshold with women more sensitive to balloon distention;
- women have a higher sphincter tone and contraction rate.

Males have greater upper esophageal sphincter axial symmetry whereas females have greater upper esophageal sphincter wet swallow after-contraction pressures upon manometry. Males normally have a longer sigmoid colon than females. Anal sphincter length and maximum squeezing pressures are larger in men. Females have a shorter anal canal and sharper colonic angulation. The normal position of the anus, defined as the ratio of the distance from the anus to the vagina or scrotum divided by the distance between the vagina or scrotum and the coccyx is 0.39 (± 0.09) in females and 0.56 (± 0.10) in males.

A female anus-fourchette: coccyx fourchette ratio of < 0.34 is abnormal. A male anus-scrotum: coccyx scrotum ratio of < 0.46 is abnormal. The puborectalis muscle represents a greater proportion of the anal canal in women (61% vs. 45%) than in men. Rectal pressures are higher in males. Women over age 60 years have more rectal compliance than men in the same age group while no difference is seen in younger persons.

The basal acid output (BAO) upper limit of normal is 10.5 mEq/h in men and 5–6 mEq/h in women. After stimulation, maximal acid output (MAO) is 5.0–30.2 mEq/h in females and 6.9–47.8 mEq/h in males. The upper limit of normal of BAO/MAO ratio is 0.23 for females and 0.29 for males. Adult males secrete more acid in their stomach than adult females. Normal adult females secrete less gastric acid than men do and men have more physiologic reflux than women.

The livers of males express twice the amount of P glycoprotein as females. This suggests that males may transport drugs out of the hepatocytes more rapidly. Nonhemoglobin iron content of the liver is 250 mg in men and 80 mg in women. In the liver, the activity of phosphoenolpyruvate carboxykinase is higher in males. Pyruvate kinases activity is higher in the liver of males.

The ratio of secondary to primary bile acids is greater in the bile of women. This may be due to the higher intracolonic pH and longer bowel transit time in women. Daily bilirubin production is lower in females. Inorganic phosphate Pi-class glutathione S-transferase is about 1.6 times greater in females' colons than in males.

Men are less sensitive to balloon distention in the esophagus, duodenum, jejunum, ileum, colon and rectum than women. The transit time from the mouth to rectal passage has been reported to be 66 hours (34–117) for men and 82 hours (47–128) for women. Females empty both solids and liquids from the gastric tract slower than men. The gastric, small intestinal and colonic mean transit times are longer in females. In the early follicular phase of menses, women have higher pressures and shorter intervals of migrating motor complexes in the jejunum than men. Phase III contraction amplitude and propagation velocity differ by gender for the jejunal migrating motor complex with the propagation velocity slower and the amplitude higher in females compared to males. Males have an average of 0.96 motions per 24 hours and women have an average of 1.16 motions per 24 hours. Males average 28 hours between motions, females 23 hours. Weight of individual stools is 142 grams for men and 111 grams for women.

Gastroenterology Laboratory Values:

Aspartate Aminotransferase
    Female: 0.15–0.42 ukat/liter
    Male: 0.17–0.67 ukat/liter

γ-Glutamyltransferase
    Male: 1–94 U/liter
    Female: 1–70 U/liter

Alkaline Phosphotase (Adults)
    Female: 0.5–1.67 ukat/liter
    Male: 0.75–1.92 ukat/liter

Alanine Aminotransferase
    Female: 0.12–0.50 ukat/liter
    Male: 0.17–0.92 ukat/liter

Ferritin
    Male: 30–300 ug/liter
    Female: 10–200 ug/liter

Diseases

Abdominal Pain
    Female > Male
    24.4% of adult females vs. 17.5% of adult males during the last month reported abdominal pain.
    The incidence is slightly > 10% in pediatric populations with a girl-boy ratio of 4:3.

Acute Intermittent Porphyria
    Female > Male (3:2)
    Typically the age of symptom development is in the 20's for females and 30's for men.

Adenocarcinoma of the Esophagus
    Male > Female
    White > Black

Adenocarcinoma of the Gallbladder
    Female > Male (2:1)

Agenesis of Abdominal Musculature
    Males > Females
    Often associated with undescended testicles in males.

Alcohol Induced Steatohepatitis
    Female gender is an independent risk factor for progression to cirrhosis.

Alcoholic Liver Disease
    Male > Female (3:1)

Alpha 1-Antitrypsin Deficiency
    Male = Female
    But liver disease progresses with age, especially in males.
    Male preponderance is between age 5–16 years, when the incidence of liver disease increases to 15%.
    Liver cancer is rare in females with alpha 1-antitrypsin deficiency but an increased incidence reported in males.
    Men are more likely to have emphysema.

Amebic Liver Abscess
    Male > Female (9–10:1)

Ampulla Tumors of the Pancreas
    Male > Female (1.5:1)

Amyand's Hernia
    Male > Female (slightly)

Anal Canal Tumor
    Female > Male (4:3)

Anal Cancer
    Female > Male
    Epidermoid cancer of anus has strong female predominance.

Anal Fissure
    Male > Female
    Females more likely to have anterior midline fissure than males (10:1).

Anal Fistulae-Idiopathic
    Male > Female (1.8–9:1)
    More striking in neonates and infants, where males predominate and have multiple fistulae compared to females. Females tend not to develop fistulae before age 2 and tend to have milder disease.

Anal Margin Tumor
    Male > Female (4:1)

Anorectal Abscess
    Male > Female (4:1)

Anorectal Fistula
    Male = Female
    Pediatric ages: Boys > Girls

Appendicitis
    Male > Female (slightly)
        Overall
    Male > Female (3:2)
        Ages 10–30 years
    Male = Female
        Over age 30 years

Autoimmune Hepatitis
    Female > Male (4:1)

Barrett's Esophagus
    Male > Female (2–4:1)
    Primarily in white males.
    Levels of Hsp27 (heat shock protein that may be protective) are higher in the esophagus of women.

Bezoars
    Female > Male (9:1)

Bile Duct Injury
    Male > Female
    Usually associated with cholecystectomy.

Biliary Atresia
    Female > Male (1.4:1)

Biliary Cyst
    Female > Male (3–8:1)

Bloating and Distension
    Female > Male
    In a survey 19.2% of women and 10.5% of men complained of these symptoms during the last month.

Boerhaave's Syndrome
    Male > Female (2–5:1)
    Esophageal perforation occurs on the right side in neonates and on the left side (90%) in adults.

Bulimia-Type Factitious Diarrhea
    Female > Male

Canker Sore
    Female > Male

Carcinoid Tumor of Appendix
Female > Male

Cathartic Colon
Female > Male (9:1)
Results from abuse of laxatives to achieve regular bowel function.

Cavernous Hemangioma of the Liver
Female > Male (4–6:1)

Cecal Volvulus
Female > Male (1.5–7:1)

Celiac Sprue
Female > Male (2:1)

Ceroid Histiocytosis of the Spleen
Male > Female

Childhood Duodenal Ulcer
Male > Female (3:1)

Cholangiocarcinoma
Male > Female (3:2)

Cholangiocarcinoma of the Extrahepatic Biliary Tract
Male > Female (slightly)

Cholangitis
Female > Male
Secondary to gall stones.
Male > Female
Secondary to malignant obstruction and HIV infection.

Cholecystitis
Female > Male (2:1)
The serum ascorbic acid level is inversely related to the prevalence of gallbladder disease (clinical and asymptomatic) in women but not in men.

Choledochal Cyst
Female > Male (3:1)
Occurs primarily in Asians.

Choledocholithiasis
Female > Male

Cholelithiasis
  Female > Male (2:1)
  In infants, Male > Female, but the incidence rises in puberty in females whereas it is negligible in males.

Chronic Active Hepatitis
  Female > Male (8:1)

Chronic Arteriosclerotic Mesenteric Vascular Occlusive Disease
  Female > Male

Chronic Constipation
  Female > Male

Chronic Diarrhea
  Female > Male

Chronic Liver Disease
  Male > Female
  Hospitalization rate: Male 33.1 per 100 thousand, female 23.9 per 100 thousand.
  Death Rate—Male 14.7 per 100 thousand, Female 6.6 per 100 thousand.

Chronic Varioliform Gastritis
  Male > Female

Cirrhosis
  Male cirrhotics undergoing surgery appear to have more complications than female cirrhotics undergoing surgery.

Collagenous Colitis
  Female > Male (10–20:1)

Colon Adenoma
  Male > Female
  Colorectal adenomas occur more in males but the malignancy rate may be higher in females.
  If one adenoma is present the risk of developing a metachronous adenoma is greater in males.

Colorectal Cancer
  Male > Female (1.3:1)
  3rd leading cancer killer in men and 2nd leading cancer killer in women.

Right sided tumors are more common in women and left sided tumors are more common in men.
The prognosis is better in women, especially parous women.
Cancer of the cecum and ascending colon is higher in females by 10–20% at all ages.

Congenital Diaphragmatic Hernia
    Male > Female (1.25:1)
        Overall
    Male > Female (slightly)
        Bochdalek
    Female > Male
        Morgagni
    Occurs on the left side in 88% of cases.

Congenital Megacolon
    Male > Female (4:1)
        Short segment
        For short segment: If male sibling affected, female has a 0.6% risk of disease.
    Male > Female (5:4)
        Long segment
        For long segment: Sibling risk if female affected, male has 18% risk of disease.

Congenital Pyloric Stenosis
    Male > Female

Constipation
    Female > Male (2–3:1)
    Women with severe constipation outnumber men (10:1)

Crohn's Disease
    Female > Male (slightly)
        Overall
    Female > Male (2:1)
        In elderly
    The lag time between bowel resection and recurrence of symptoms is shorter in females (4.8 vs. 6.5 years).
    Female patients are more likely to have relatives with Crohn's disease than male patients.
    Ileocecal resection appears to be more common in females.

Smoking adversely affects the clinical course of the disease more so in females.

Cronkhite-Canada Syndrome
Male > Female (3:2)

Cystadenoma of Pancreas
Female > Male

Cystosarcoma Phyllodes
Female > Male

Diarrhea, Chronic
Female > Male

Diverticula of Intestine
Female > Male (2:1)

Duodenal Diverticula
Female > Male (2:1)

Duodenal Ulcer
Male > Female (2:1)
Mortality: Male > Female
Postprandial gastrin concentrations are higher in female patients with duodenal ulcers.

Dyskeratosis Congenita
Male > Female

Encopresis
Male > Female (1.5–3:1)

Epigastric Hernia
Male > Female

Esophageal Atresia and Tracheoesophageal Fistula
Male > Female (1.26:1)

Esophageal Cancer
Male > Female (2.6–3:1)
Survival is higher in women for adenocarcinoma and squamous cell carcinoma.

Esophageal Varices
Male > Female

Esophageal Web
    Female > Male

Esophagitis
    Female > Male

Familial Adenomatous Polyposis
    In some studies the onset of symptoms and colorectal cancer is earlier in females.

Fatty Liver
    Male > Female

Fecal Impaction
    Male > Female
    No sex preponderance in adults but in children, 75% are male.

Fecal Incontinence
    Female > Male

Femoral Hernia
    Female > Male
            Adult
    Female = Male
            Child

Fibrolamellar Carcinoma of Liver
    Female > Male (1–2:1)

Focal Nodular Hyperplasia of the Liver
    Female > Male (2:1)

Functional Bowel Disease
    Female > Male (20:1)
    For unexplained GI tract symptoms.

Functional Dyspepsia
    Female > Male

Gallbladder Cancer
    Female > Male (2–4:1)
    In part due to the higher incidence of gallstones in females.

Gallstones
    Female > Male (2–3:1)
    Ratio difference reflects cholesterol stones (7:4) female to male.

20–25% of females over age 55 years have gallstones.
10% of males over age 55 have gallstones.
In some countries gender ratio is (1:1) reflecting a predominance of pigmented stones.
Cholesterol stones account for 85% of gallstones in the U.S.
Endogenous estrogens increase biliary cholesterol secretion, offering an explanation for increased risk of cholesterol gallstone formation in females and progesterone inhibits gallbladder emptying. After menopause, females lose their increased risk for gallstone formation.

Gastric Cancer
Male > Female (3:2)
Early menopause predisposes women to gastric cancer.
Helicobacter pylori bacteria may be associated with a higher incidence of gastric cancer in females in some studies.

Gastric and Gastroepiploic Artery Aneurysm
Male > Female (3:1)

Gastric Hemangioma
Male > Female

Gastric Leiomyosarcoma
Male > Female (2:1)

Gastric Lipoma
Male > Female

Gastric Lymphoma
Male > Female

Gastric Paresis due to Diabetes Mellitus
Female > Male (8–9:1)

Gastric Ulcer
Male > Female (2.3:1.8)
Mortality: Male > Female
Females predominate among nonsteroidal anti-inflammatory drug users that develop ulcers.

Gastroesophageal Reflux Disease
Female > Male (slightly)
NHANES 2 found GERD in 3.18% of females and 2.94% of males.

The mean basal level of acid output is higher in males than females. Men have more serious forms of the disease (ulcers and strictures). Asymptomatic males have more acid exposure and wider variability than asymptomatic females on esophageal pH monitoring. Males have more physiologic reflux than females.

Gilbert's Disease (Syndrome)
 Male > Female (3:1)

Glossitis
 Male > Female

Glucagonoma
 Female > Male (4:1)

Granular Cell Tumor of the Gallbladder
 Female > Male

Growth Hormone Releasing Factor Tumor
 Female > Male (3:1)

Heartburn
 Female > Male

Hemochromatosis
 Male = Females
 But Male > Female (8:1) for clinical signs.

Hepatic Adenoma
 Female > Male (3–4:1)
 Primarily in females on oral contraceptives.

Hepatic Artery Aneurysm
 Male > Female (2:1)

Hepatic Focal Nodular Hyperplasia
 Female > Male

Hepatic Hemangioma
 Female > Male

Hepatic Tumor
 Large cavernous hemangioma
  More common in females.
 Liver cell adenoma
  More common in females (90%).

Hepatitis B, Chronic
: Females are more likely to respond to interferon therapy.

Hepatitis B, Fulminant
: Male > Female (2:1)

Hepatitis C
: Male > Female (2:1)

Hepatitis, Chronic Active Autoimmune
: Female > Male (8:1)

Hepatoblastoma
: Male > Female

Hepatocellular Adenoma
: Female > Male
: Primarily in females taking birth control pills.

Hepatocellular Carcinoma
: Male > Female (3–8:1)

Hepatoma
: Male > Female (3–4:1)

Hepatorenal Syndrome
: Male > Female

Hernia, Inguinal
: Male > Female
: Indirect inguinal hernia is the most common hernia in men and women. 25% of males and 2% of females will develop inguinal hernia during their lifetime.
: Hernias occur more on the right side than the left.

Hernia, Sliding Hiatal
: Female > Male (4:1)

Hiccups
: Male > Female (4:1)

Hirschsprung's Disease
: Male > Female (3.8:1)
: : Limited disease (rectosigmoid)
: Male > Female (2.2:1)
: : Total Colonic Agangliosis

Hypertrophic Pyloric Stenosis
    Male > Female (2.5–5.5:1)
    40% of patients needing surgery for HPS are firstborn males.
    There is a higher rate of HPS in children of women who have had surgery for HPS than in children of men operated on for this condition (20% vs. 5%).

Idiopathic Acid Hypersecretion
    Male > Female (4:1)

Idiopathic Aconatal Hepatitis
    Male > Female

Idiopathic Chronic Pancreatitis (Juvenile Form)
    Male > Female

Idiopathic Chronic Ulcerative Enteritis
    Female > Male (slightly)

Immunoproliferative Small Intestinal Disease
    Male > Female

Imperforate Anus
    Male > Female (2:1)
        High lesion
    Male = Female
        Low lesion

Incontinence, Anal
    Female > Male

Infantile Hypertrophic Pyloric Stenosis
    Male > Female (4–5:1)
    HPS develops in 19% of male offspring and 7% of female offspring born to mothers with HPS.
    About 5% of boys and 2.5% of girls with pyloric stenosis were born to fathers who had HPS.

Inflammatory Bowel Disease
    Females have higher levels of symptom severity and rating of inflammatory bowel disease (IBD) concerns than men.
    Patient concerns that differ by gender include attractiveness, intimacy and sexual performance. Women also have more concerns about self-image, feel more alone and more fearful of having children.

The onset of menses may be delayed in girls that develop IBS before or during puberty.

Active Crohn's disease may impair fertility in women.

Women with ulcerative colitis are at no greater risk for early menopause but women with Crohn's disease may enter menopause earlier.

The incidence of osteoporosis is higher in women with IBD than in women without IBD.

Intraductal Papilloma of Pancreas
Male > Female (2:1)

Better prognosis than ductal adenocarcinoma.

Intrarectal Prolapse
Female > Male (4:1)

Intussusception
Male > Female (3:2)

Male predominance is more notable in older infants.

Irritable Bowel Syndrome
Female > Male (2–6:1)
    In the United States
Male > Female
    In other countries

In one study, 53% of females had a history of abuse.

Aloestron is an effective treatment in females with diarrhea predominant IBS but not in males.

Male patients have elevated baseline and stimulated sympathetic outflow to the heart and skin.

Women have slower whole gut transit time than men, and report more constipation and more sensitivity to pain than men.

Females are more likely to complain of constipation, abdominal distension and of certain extracolonic symptoms.

Isolated Nonspecific Ulcer of the Small Intestine
Male > Female (slightly)

Juvenile Intestinal Polyps
Male > Female

Kohlmeier-Degos Syndrome
Male > Female

Laxative Abuse
　　Female > Male

Leukoplakia, Oral
　　Male > Female

Liver Abscess, Pyogenic
　　Male > Female (slightly)

Liver Cyst (Solitary Nonparasitic)
　　Female > Male (4:1)

Liver Disease
　　Alcoholic
　　　　Females are more susceptible to alcohol induced liver injury. It requires less alcohol per day to cause liver injury in females.
　　　　Women have a decreased concentration of alcohol dehydorgenase in the stomach.
　　　　Females may be more likely to progress to cirrhosis than men.
　　Hemochromatosis
　　　　Male > Female
　　　　Clinical disease more apparent in males.
　　　　Whites > Blacks
　　Primary Biliary Cirrhosis
　　　　Female > Male
　　　　90% are female.
　　Hepatitis B
　　　　Risk of infection seems higher if infected partner is male.
　　Autoimmune Hepatitis
　　　　Female > Male
　　　　Females make up 80% of cases.
　　　　Type 2 autoimmune hepatitis occurs most often in adolescence or young females. This type is very aggressive and may lead to fulminant hepatitis.

Mallory-Weiss Tear
　　Male > Female (4:1)

Meckel's Diverticulum
　　Male > Female (1.6–3:1)
　　　　Overall

Most frequent congenital anomaly of the GI tract.
Males are more likely to become symptomatic than females (2.7:1).
Complications occur more frequently in males.
Male = Female
    Asymptomatic disease:

Mediterranean Abdominal Lymphoma
    Male > Female

Menetrier's Disease
    Male > Female

Mesenteric Venous Thrombosis
    Male > Female (slightly)

Nausea
    Female > Male

Nitrofurantoin Induced Chronic Hepatitis
    Female > Male (9:1)

Nonalcoholic Steatohepatitis Syndrome
    Female > Male
    Primarily in middle age obese females with Type 2 diabetes.

Nonalcoholic Steatosis
    Female > Male
    Especially in obese women.
    Also occurs in men who are as little as 10% overweight.

Nonulcer Dyspepsia
    Female > Male

Obesity
    Female > Male
    Occurs in 20–30% of adult men, 30–40% of adult women.

Ogilvie's Syndrome
    Males present in their 7th decade, females present at an earlier age.

Oral Cavity Cancer
    Male > Female
    Accounts for 4% of cancer in men, 2% in women.

Oral Leukoplakia
    Male > Female

Oral Lichen Planus
   Female > Male

Pancreatic Adenocarcinoma
   Male > Female (slightly)

Pancreatic Cancer
   Male > Female (1.5–2.1:1)
   Mean age in males is 63 years.
   Mean age in females is 67 years.
   Solid and Papillary neoplasms of pancreas are more common in females.
   Females have a slightly longer survival.

Pancreatic and Pancreaticoduodenal and Gastroduodenal Artery Aneursym
   Male > Female (4:1)

Pancreatitis, Chronic
   Male > Female (2–5:1)

Paraumbilical Hernia
   Female > Male (5:1)

Peptic Ulcer Disease
   Male > Female (slightly)
      Duodenal Ulcer: Lifetime prevalence: 10% male, 5% female.
      Upper GI bleeding from peptic ulcer is twice as likely in males.
   Male > Female
      Recurrence of PUD
   Male > Female
      Gastric Ulcer
      Female predominance with NSAID use.
      The number of deaths from bleeding gastric ulcer is higher in females (10.5% vs. 8.7%).

Perirectal Abscess
   Male > Female

Peritonitis, Acute
   Male > Female

Peritonitis, Spontaneous Bacterial
　　Male > Female

Pilonidal Disease
　　Male > Female (2–10:1)

Plummer Vinson Syndrome
　　Female > Male

Polyps in the Distal Colon
　　Males are 3.3 times as likely to have proximal neoplasms as females compared to people without distal polyps.

Porphyria Cutanea Tarda
　　Male > Female
　　Especially seen in alcoholics.

Portal Hypertension
　　Male > Female

Postprandial Fullness
　　Female > Male

Primary Biliary Cirrhosis
　　Female > Male (9–10:1)
　　Males tend to have higher serum alkaline phosphatase levels and lower frequency of occurrence of piecemeal necrosis.

Primary Gastric Lymphoma
　　Male > Female (2:1)

Primary Peritonitis
　　Female > Male
　　Thought to be due to introduction of bacteria through fallopian tubes.

Primary Sclerosing Cholangitis
　　Male > Female (3–3.5:2)

Proctalgia Fugax
　　Female > Male

Proctitis
　　Male > Female

Pruritus Ani
    Male > Female (4:1)

Pyloric Stenosis
    Male > Female (5:1)
    Occurs in 1/150 male live births, 1/750 female live births.

Pyogenic Liver Abscess
    Male = Female
        Overall
    Female > Male
        From biliary tract disease.

Pyogenic Liver Abscess (Cryptogenic)
    Male > Female

Rectal Cancer
    Male > Female (5:3)

Rectal Prolapse
    Female > Male (5–9:1)
    Slight male predominance in children.

Retractile Mesenteritis
    Male > Female (2:1)

Salivary Gland Calculi
    Male > Female (slightly)

Salivary Gland Tumors
    Female > Male
        Pleomorphic adenoma
    Male = Female
        Other adenomas

Sigmoid Volvulus
    Female > Male (2–3:1)

Small Bowel Lipoma
    Male > Female

Small Bowel Tumor, Malignant
    Male > Female (slightly)

Solitary Rectal Ulcer Syndrome
    Female > Male (2:1)

Spastic Esophageal Disorder
    Female > Male

Sphincter of Oddi Dysfunction
    Female > Male

Splenic Artery Aneurysm
    Female > Male (4:1)

Squamous Cell Cancer of the Esophagus
    Male > Female
    Black > White

Stomach Cancer
    Male > Female (11:7)

Superior Mesenteric Artery Syndrome
    Female > Male (2:1)
    Average age in females 41 years; in males 38 years.

Tongue and Lip Tumors
    Male > Female

Tracheoesophageal Fistula
    Male > Female

Transverse and Splenic Flexure Volvulus
    Female > Male

Umbilical Hernia
    Female > Male

Vasoactive Intestinal Polypeptide Tumors
    Female > Male (3:1)

Whipple's Disease
    Male > Female (9:1)
    Symptoms of arthritis often precede diagnosis by an average of 9 years.

Wilson's Disease, Fulminant
    Female > Male
    The His1069Gln mutation is more common in females.
    Female hormones may aggravate hepatic copper accumulation.

Zollinger-Ellison Syndrome
   Male > Female (3:2)
   Females are more likely to have malignant course.

Orthopedics/Rheumatology

Anatomy and Physiology

Bone accretion occurs during adolescence when there is a large increase in bone mass. Over a lifetime women lose approximately 50% of their trabecular bone and 30% of their cortical bone whereas men lose two thirds of this amount. In male cortical bone, bone resorption occurs resulting in cortical thinning; however a simultaneous increase occurs in periosteal locations. But in females undergoing endocortical thinning, the same periosteal bone gain is not seen. In trabecular bone, the male trabecular plate thinning and dropout occurs the same as in females. Bone mineral density (BMD) is greater in males and the rate of decline in BMD with age is slower in males. Female bones are usually smaller and more slender than male equivalents, i.e. smaller shaft diameter relative to length. Females show earlier ossification and epiphyseal fusion than males, a difference which is presumably genetic. Sexual differences are marked in the pelvis and skull, but not equally so in all populations. Females in general have shorter limbs relative to body length, especially in the arms. The humerus, but not the forearm, is shorter in females than males. Women also have a narrower shoulder girdle and increased ligamentous laxity of the shoulder. The legs of males comprise 56% of their height but only 51% of female's height. The center of gravity is lower in females. Therefore females have an advantage in balance sports such as gymnastics.

Females have more joint hypermobility and musculotendinus flexibility than men. Joint laxity increases during pregnancy, especially in the third trimester. Laxity is increased in multigravidae versus primagravidae. The hormones estrogen and relaxin fluctuate during the menstrual cycle and are reported to increase ligamentous laxity and decrease neuromuscular performance.

In adults the average body fat content is 12–16% in males and 26% in females. The lean body weight of man is greater than woman of the same height and contains more muscle mass. Overall, the females' absolute strength and power is about 2/3rds of males. However, unit for unit female muscle tissue is similar in force output to male muscle tissue. The onset of the pubertal growth spurt precedes or is associated with early signs of sexual maturation in girls. In boys the onset of sexual maturation precedes the onset of the pubertal growth spurt. During adolescence girls do not have a significant change in muscle mass but their hips broaden relative to their shoulders. Boys undergo an increase in muscle mass, and shoulders broaden relative to hips. Androgens have greater anabolic effects on bone and muscle mass than do estrogens. Before age 11 girls are about 90% as strong as boys but this decreases to 75% at age 15–16 years. For the same mass and activity level, males require more kcal to meet daily energy requirements.

Females are more likely to have a more flexible knee joint and a smaller notch in the femur. When women flex their knees between 0–30 degrees, the femoral condyles provide less support to the patella, which is positioned more laterally in the femoral sulcus than in males.

Males have a narrower pelvis and less flexible hips, more developed thigh muscles, less flexible knee joint and wider notch in the femur, neutral or internal rotation of the tibia, neutral rotation of the femur, and genu varum compared to females. Females have a wider pelvis and greater hip varus, femoral anteversion, knee valgus, Q angle, and foot pronation than males of equal age. Females are more likely to have internal rotation of the femur, and external rotation of the tibia, and less developed thigh muscles. Females have more anterior tibial laxity, less muscular strength and endurance, and require more time to produce similar levels of muscular force. The width of the femoral intercondylar notch and the notch width index (relation of the condylar width to notch width) are less in females than in males.

Most males have an anthropoid or android pelvis, most females have an android or gynecoid pelvis. The female pelvis is lighter, the bones are more slender and the markings made by the attachments of the muscles are less pronounced; the ilium has a greater lateral flair, and the iliac fossa is slightly shallower. The pubic arch is wider in the female; the ischial spines do not project toward the center of the pelvis as they do in males and the ischial tuberosities are farther apart. In females, the inlet to the true pelvis tends to be oval rather than heart shaped, the ischial spines do not project into the outlets of the pelvis as they do in males, and the same is true of the sacrum and coccyx. All diameters in the true pelvis are longer in the female. The female sacrum is shorter and wider, producing a wider pelvic cavity. The central concavity is deeper in females and its deepest point is usually higher than in males; curvature above this point is greater in the female. The dorsal protrusion of the second sacral vertebra is therefore usually less prominent in males. In females the pelvic surface faces downwards more than in males, increasing the pelvic cavity and making the lumbosacral angle more prominent. The female auricular surface is shorter, but in both sexes usually extends along the first three sacral vertebrae. Owing to the great size of the fifth lumbar body, the first sacral body occupies a larger proportion of the sacral base in the male, its transverse diameter exceeding the length of an ala; the female dimensions are roughly equal.

Females have higher ranges of total hip motion, internal rotation, total rotation and hip abduction. The maximum eccentric and concentric peak torque of the quadriceps of the male is 8% and 23% higher respectively than in the female. Women rely more on their quadriceps and gastrocnemius muscles and less on their hamstrings than men. Female athletes tend to have weaker knee extension and flexion strength than men athletes.

In both the tibia and femur, men have larger section moduli and bone strength indices than women. Female bones are narrower and have thinner cortices. Females have greater extension at the metacarpophalangeal joints in both active and passive motion Secondary ossification centers of the hand appear earlier in girls than boys. Men show little change in cortical area and some increase in second moments of area with age while women show decrease in both cortical area and second moments of area of the lower limb bones. The distal physis of the femur fusion occurs at approximately age 15 in girls and age 17 in boys. The scapholunate distance is longer in male children than female children. Sternal length is longer in males than in females by 22 mm. Prepubertal vertebral size is 11% greater in boys than similarly matched girls. In postpuberty the cross-sectional area of the vertebra is 25% greater in men. The index finger is longer than the ring finger in the majority of females but the ring finger is longer than the index finger in the majority of males. Center of gravity of females is slightly lower than males. Females tend to have a more narrow rear foot. The shape of the trapezial bone surface in the hand is different between the sexes.

The female CMC thumb joint is less congruent than the males. Females have a greater ligamentous laxity of the lateral ankle than men. Males have more knee cartilage than females. (Males have 16–31% higher cartilage volume). Females have a greater range of motion of the cervical spine except in forward flexion.

In terms of muscle firing patterns and lower extremity muscle strength ratios, females tend to be quadriceps-dominant, that is they rely more on their quadriceps muscles than their hamstring muscles to stabilize the knee in response to anterior tibia translation. Males activate their hamstrings at three times the level of females during landing and cutting maneuvers. Females have significantly less lower extremity strength and endurance, particularly in the hamstrings. The lower body strength of the average female reaches 70% of the average male. Females perform cutting and landing maneuvers with a more erect hip-trunk posture, more knee valgus, and less knee flexion than males. Females tend to jump and land with their quadriceps muscles while men tend to use their hamstring muscles. Trunk muscle moment-arms are larger for males than females. Trunk muscle geometry of males and females are different. Females tend to have smaller muscle fiber size, less capillary supply per fiber, and a different fiber composition and metabolic profile than men. The total cross sectional area of muscles in women is 60–85% that of men. Maximum unloaded shortening velocity (VO) of Type IIA fibers is reduced in males with increasing age but not Type I fibers. But in females VO is reduced with age in Type I fibers but not Type IIA fibers. Older women have a lower VO than older men in both fiber types but no difference in young women compared to young men. The Type IIA muscle fibers are largest in men and Type I fibers largest in women in the vastus lateralis muscle. The mean cross sectional area of all fibers of the vastus lateralis muscle are smaller in females. Levels of glycolytic enzyme markers are higher in male vastus lateralis skeletal muscle. The muscle fiber-type distribution in the trapezius muscle is similar between the sexes but the cross-sectional fiber area is greater in men. In the gastrocnemius and soleus muscles, females have longer average muscle fiber bundle length but males have thicker muscles and larger angles of pennation. Females have a higher adductor pollicis muscle oxidative capacity than men and fatigue of the adductor pollicis muscle develops slower in women upon submaximal intermittent contractions.

Back extension strength (BES) peaks in the 4th decade in men and the 5th decade in women. Women's BES is 54% to 76% of men's BES.

Men have a greater loss of BES than women with increasing age. The upper body strength of the average female is about one half of the average male, although when matched for size a woman has 80% of the upper body strength. The muscle mass of females is about 23% of body weight versus 40% in males.

The serum urate concentration varies with age and sex. At puberty, serum urate concentration increases by 1–2 mg/dl in males. In contrast, females exhibit little change in their serum urate concentration until menopause, when concentrations increase to approach values seen in adult men. Studies have demonstrated that the mean clearance of uric acid was 1.2–2.3 ml/min higher in females than males

On average, males are taller than females by 12.5 cm.

Target Height of a Child
  Male = (father's height (cm) + mother's height (cm) + 13) / 2
  Female = (father's height (cm) + mother's height (cm) - 13) / 2

Sex Differences (mean) in Muscle Physiology: Control (C) vs Athlete (A)

	Male C	Male A	Female C	Female A
Anterior Tibial translation (mm)				
Relaxed	5.8	3.5	6.5	4.5
Contracted	2.8	1.8	3.0	2.4
Isokinetic Strength (% of body Weight)				
Quadriceps	88.4	82.3	72.5	76.7
Hamstrings	46.7	48.3	38.6	40.9
Isokinetic Endurance (% body weight)				
Quadriceps	39.6	40.5	31.3	35.5
Hamstrings	20.5	22.6	16.5	20.0
Time to peak torque (msec)				
Quadriceps				
60 deg/sec	463	408	448	420
240 deg/sec	150	153	170	158
Hamstrings				
60 deg/sec	443	328	426	430
240 deg/sec	170	150	164	169

Anthropometric Measurement of Americans Adults
(50th percentile values in centimeters)

Criteria	Males	Females
Heights		
Standing		
Standing Height	175.58	162.94
Eye Height	163.39	151.61
Shoulder Height	144.25	133.36
Elbow Height	107.25	99.79
Wrist Height	84.65	79.03
Crotch Height	83.72	77.14
Sitting		
Sitting Height (normal)	99.39	85.20
Eye Height	79.20	73.87
Shoulder Height	59.78	55.55
Elbow Height	23.06	22.05
Thigh Height	16.82	15.89
Knee Height	55.88	51.54
Popliteal Height	43.41	38.94
Depths		
Forward Reach	80.08	73.46
Buttock-Knee Distance (sitting)	61.64	58.89
Buttock-Popliteal Distance (sitting)	50.04	48.17
Elbow-Fingertip Distance	48.40	44.29
Chest Depth	24.32	23.94
Breadths		
Forearm-Forearm	54.61	46.85
Hip (sitting)	36.68	38.45
Head Dimensions		
Circumference	56.77	54.62
Breadth	15.17	14.44
Interpupillary Breadth	6.47	6.06
Hand Dimensions		
Circumference (metacarpal)	21.38	18.62

Hand Length	19.38	18.05
Hand Breadth (metacarpal)	9.04	7.94
Thumb Breadth	2.41	2.07
Foot Dimensions		
Foot Length	26.97	24.44
Foot Breadth	10.06	8.97
Lateral Malleolus Height	6.71	6.06
Weight	166 pounds	137 pounds

Lumbar Spine Compressive Strength (kN)
    Female: 3.97 ± 1.50
    Male: 5.81 ± 2.58

Diseases

Females are more likely to suffer than males from many common musculoskeletal disorders, more likely to be hospitalized for these disorders, and the average length of hospital stay is longer.

Achilles Tendon Rupture
    Male > Female

Acne Conglobota
    Male > Female (4:1)
    Musculoskeletal manisfestations occur usually in black men.

Acute Calcific Periarthritis of the Finger Joint and Large Toe
    Female > Male
    Due to apatite crystal deposition.

Adamantinoma
    Male > Female

Adhesive Capsulitis of the Shoulder
    Female > Male (2:1)

Adolescent Idiopathic Scoliosis
    Female = Male
    But, females are more likely to need treatment.

Adult Onset Still's Disease
    Female > Male

Alkaptonuria
  Female = Male
  Arthritis is worse in men.

Allergic Granulomatosis and Angiitis
  Male > Female
  52–65% of cases occur in males.

Amyloidosis
  Male > Female (2:1)

Ankle Sprain
  Female > Male

Ankylosing Spondylitis
  Male > Female (3–10:1)
  Females tend to have a milder disease (and possibly a frequency approaching men in some studies) with fewer spinal problems but more knee and ankle joint involvement.
  Axial disease appears to be more severe in males.
  Females may be 2 times as likely to pass the disease on to their children as men. The children of women with AS before age 21 years were 7 times more likely to get AS than were children of men diagnosed at a young age. The prevalence of AS among the relatives of women with the disease did not differ significantly by sex. In contrast, the male relatives of men with AS were more than twice as likely to develop the disease as were the female relatives.

Anserine Bursitis
  Female > Male

Anterior Cruciate Ligament Injuries
  Female > Male (4–8:1)
  Females often perform athletic maneuvers with greater extension and quadriceps activation.
  Rates of ACL injuries may vary in women according to the menstrual cycle phase. More ACL injuries occur during the ovulatory phase than the follicular phase. Levels of estrogen and relaxin are elevated during ovulation.
  Most experts feel the female's wider hips puts more stress on the ACL. The wider pelvic dimension in females produces increased external tibial torsion and excessive subtalar joint pronation causing an increased thigh-foot angle.

Females also have increased valgus angle, relatively less muscle mass and strength, variation in the intercondylar notch dimensions and ligament size and increased collagen laxity.

After reconstructive surgery for ACL tears, return of strength, proprioception, and control may be slower in females.

ACL injuries tend to be more severe in females and more likely to require surgery.

Antiphospholipid Antibody Syndrome
Female > Male (7–9:1–3)

Arthritis Robustus
Male > Female

Arthroplasty
Although females have a higher rate of arthritis of the knees and hips, they are less likely to undergo arthroplastic surgery than men.

Articular Infections in Rheumatoid Arthritis
Male > Female

Autoimmune Diseases
Female > Male
It's the 10th leading cause of death in every age category of women < 65 years old.
Females are more likely to develop a TH1 response after challenge with an infection or antigen, except during pregnancy, than are men.
Immune responses tend to be more vigorous in females resulting in greater antibody production and increased cell-mediated immunity after immunization; sex hormones play some role.
During pregnancy, rheumatoid arthritis and multiple sclerosis decrease in disease severity whereas lupus often worsens.
Females with autoimmune arthritis tend to get more joint pain and loss of mobility than do men.

Avascular Necrosis of the Femoral Head
Male > Female

Behcet's Disease
Male > Female
More severe in males.
66% of cases occur in males.

Benign Hypermobility Syndrome
  Female > Male
  Seen usually in preadolescent and adolescent gymnasts.

Blastomycosis Arthritis
  Male > Female

Bunionettes
  Female > Male

Bunions
  Female > Male (10–15:1)

Bursitis
  Males > Females

Bypass Arthritis Dermatitis Syndrome
  Female > Male (3:1)

Calcaneal Apophysitis
  Male > Female
  Primarily in children between 7–12 years of age.

Calcific Tendonitis
  Female > Male

Capomelia Dysplasia
  Female > Male

Carpal Boss
  Female > Male

Carpal Tunnel Syndrome
  Female > Male (3–6:1)
  More common in elderly females.

Causalgia Syndrome
  Male > Female

Cervical Hyperextension Injuries
  Male > Female

Cervical Spine Injury
  Male > Female

Cervical Spondylosis
  Male > Female (3:2)

Cervical Strain Injury, Sports-related
    Female > Male

Charcot Joint
    Male > Female

Chilblains
    Female > Male

Chondrodysplasia Punctata, X-Linked
    Female > Male
    Usually fatal in males.

Chondromalacia Patellae
    Female > Male

Chondrosarcoma
    Male > Female (3:2)

Chordoma
    Male > Female (5:3)
    Females are more likely to present with cranial involvement, men with sacral involvement.

Chronic Active Liver Disease
    Female > Male

Chronic Fatigue Syndrome
    Female > Male (1.3–4:1)
    95% of cases are white.
    Women report more sore throat, painful lymph nodes, morning stiffness, and irritable bowel syndrome. Physical functioning is reported as worse among women.
    Lifetime diagnosis of somatization is more common in women.

Chronic Joint Symptoms, Activity Limitation
    Female > Male

Chronic Recurrent Multifocal Osteitis
    Female > Male (2:1)

Churg-Strauss Syndrome
    Male > Female (2:1)

Clubfoot
    Male > Female (2:1)

Bilateral in 30–50% of cases.
Risk of having a subsequent child with clubfoot if the first child is a boy is 1 in 40, but if the first child is a girl, the risk is 1 in 16.

Coccygodynia
Female > Male

Complex Regional Pain Syndrome
Female > Male

Condensing Osteitis of Clavicles
Female > Male

Congenital Clubfoot
Male > Female

Congenital Dislocation of Hip
Female > Male (6:1)

Congenital Hip Dysplasia
Female > Male

Costochondritis
Female > Male

CPPD Disease
Male > Female (1.4:1)
Calcium pyrophosphate dihydrate crystal deposition

CREST Syndrome
Female > Male (8.5:1)

Cryoglobulinemic Vasculitis
Female > Male (2–3:1)

Cutaneous Lupus Erythematosus
Female > Male
Acute
Female > Male (2.5:1)
Subacute
Female > Male (3:1)
Chronic

Degenerative Scoliosis
Female > Male (2:1)

Degenerative Spondylolisthesis
    Female > Male (6:1)

Dequervain's Syndrome
    Female > Male (10:1)

Dermatomyositis
    Female > Male (2.5:1)
        Adults
        15–20% of patients over age 50 years have associated malignancy.
    Female = Male
        Children

Developmental Dysplasia of Hip
    Female > Male (6:1)
    Occurs in 1 in 600 females, 1 in 4000 males.
    Occurs on the left side in 60%, right side in 20% and bilaterally in 20% of cases.
    White > Black (30:1)
    Rare in Asian children.

DISH (Diffuse Idiopathic Skeletal Hyperostosis) Syndrome
    Male > Female (2:1)

Drug Induced Systemic Lupus Erythematosus
    Male > Female

Dupuytren's Contracture
    Male > Female (2–10:1)
    White > Black

Ehlers-Danlos Syndrome IX
    Male > Female

Eosinophilic Fasciitis
    Male > Female (2:1)
    Often precipitated by heavy exercise.

Epidermal Inclusion Cyst of Hand/Wrist
    Male > Female

Erdheim-Chester Disease
    Male > Female (1.6:1)

Erythema Nodusum
    Female > Male (3:1)

Ewing's Sarcoma
    Male > Female (1.9:1.2)

Fabry Disease
    Male > Female

Familial Mediterranean Fever
    Male > Female
    Occurs primarily in East Mediterranean ethnic groups.

Felty's Syndrome
    Female > Male (6.5:3.5)

Femoral Neck Fracture
    Female > Male (3:1)

Fibroma of Tendon Sheath
    Male > Female (3:1)

Fibromyalgia
    Female > Male (8–9:1)
    Tenderness is more prominent in females. In one study, 25% of females vs. 7% of males had tender points.
    Women often have more fatigue, irritable bowel syndrome, and more tender points and "pain all over".
    Women are 10 times as likely to have more than 11 tender points compared to men.
    Women are more likely to report relief of pain with local heat.
    Men with fibromyalgia report more severe symptoms, greater pain, decreased physical function, and lower quality of life.

Fibrosarcoma of the Soft Tissue
    Male > Female

Fibrositis
    Female > Male

Fibrous Dysplasia of the Bone
    Female > Male

Orthopedics/Rheumatology 209

Foot Pain
> Female > Male (2:1)
> Over 90% of foot surgery is performed on females.

Forearm Fracture
> Female > Male
> The lifetime risk is 2.5% in males and 16% in females.

Fracture
> Female > Male
> The lifetime risk of fractures at all sites is three times higher in women. The lifetime risk for any type of fracture is 40% in females vs. 13% for males. 20% of hip fractures occur in men.
> Adolescent boys and young adult males sustain more fractures than girls and young adult females probably because young males are involved in more activities that can cause skeletal trauma. After middle age, women predominate, which is felt to be due to the effects of estrogen deficiency on the bones.

Friebergs Disease
> Female > Male (3:1)

Frozen Shoulder
> Female > Male

Ganglia
> Female > Male (3:1)

Giant Cell Arteritis
> Female > Male (2–3:1)
> About 20% of cases are in males.

Giant Cell Tumor of the Bone
> Male > Female

Giant Cell Tumor of Hand/Wrist
> Male > Female (3:2)

Glomus Tumor
> Female > Male (2:1)

Gout
> Male > Female (20:1)
> Rare in females before menopause.
> Almost all acute attacks before age 50 years occur in males.

Hyperuricemia may be an indication of potential risk of hypertension for adolescent males.

Urate levels increase in males during puberty to adult levels. In contrast, urate levels remain constant in females until menopause. Females have more tophi.

Greater Trochanteric Bursitis
Female > Male

Greenstick Fracture
In girls, it is less likely to spontaneously correct than in boys.

Hallux Valgus
Female > Male

Hammertoe
Female > Male

Hemochromatosis
Male > Female (10:1)
Symptomatic

Hemophilic Arthropathy
Male > Female

Hip Fracture
Female > Male (2–3:1)
Consequences of hip fracture worse for elderly men. The death rate within 1 year of hip fracture is 26% higher for men. The incidence is rising in both sexes.

The estimated lifetime risk of hip fracture is 6% in men but up to 17.5% in white women.

Hypergammaglobulinenic Purpura of Waldenstrom
Female > Male

Hypocomplementemic Vasculitis
Female > Male

Idiopathic Osteonecrosis of Tarsal Navicular
Male > Female

Iliotibial Friction Syndrome
Female > Male

Inclusion Body Myositis
　Male > Female (3:1)

Increased PRPP Synthetase Activity
　Male > Female

Inflammatory Myopathies
　Female > Male (2:1)
　　Overall
　Male > Female (2:1)
　　Inclusion body myositis

Isolated Angiitis of the Central Nervous System
　Male > Female (slightly)

Juvenile Spondyloarthropathies
　Male > Female (2–7:1)
　　Juvenile Ankylosing Spondylitis
　Female > Male (1.6:1)
　　Juvenile Dermatomyositis
　Female > Male (2:1)
　　Juvenile Rheumatoid Arthritis
　　A risk for chronic uveitis in young girls and axial skeletal involvement in older boys. Uveitis is more likely to occur in girls with oligoarthritis of an early onset and who are ANA seropositive.
　　　Polyarticular: Rhematoid factor positive
　　　　Female > Male (8:1)
　　　Polyarticular: Rheumatoid factor negative
　　　　Female > Male (6:1).
　　　Pauciarticular, young age onset
　　　　Female > Male (7–8:1)
　　　　Girls with the HLA-A2 gene are at increased risk of developing pauciarticular JRA but the risk for boys with A2 gene is low.
　　　Pauciarticular, older age onset
　　　　Male > Female (10:1)
　　　Systemic onset (Still's Disease)
　　　　Male > Female (5:4)
　Female > Male (2:1)
　　Juvenile Psoriatic

Male > Female (4:1)
    Juvenile Reiter's
Female > Male (4.3:1)
    Juvenile SLE

Kawasaki's Disease
    Male > Female (1.3–1.5:1)
    Males are more likely to develop coronary aneurysms.
    60% of cases are male.

Kienbock's Disease
    Male > Female

Knee Arthritis
    Female > Male (1.5–2:1)
    Females are less likely to get arthroplasty but the need is as great as or greater than males.
    Females have more pain and disability than men at the time of arthroplasty.

Knee Injury
    Female athletes have a 4 to 6 fold higher incidence than males.
    High school females have nearly 5 times the incidence of knee surgery as high school males.
    Female athletes have 2 to 8 times as many anterior cruciate ligament tears.

Knee Pain
    Female > Male
    Among adults > 60 years of age, 23.5% of women and 18.1% of men complain of chronic knee pain.
    Nearly two thirds of all total knee replacements are performed on women.
    Frequency of knee pain in females begins to exceed males starting in the 20+ year old range.

Kohler's Disease I
    Male > Female

Legg-Calve-Perthes Disease
    Male > Female (4:1)
        Overall
    Male > Female (7:1)

Bilateral cases
Females seem to have more severe involvement.

Linear Scleroderma
Female > Male (3:1)

Livedoid Vasculitis
Female > Male

Lipoma Arborescens
Male > Female

Lipoma of Hand/Wrist
Female > Male (slightly)

Localized Nodular Tenosynovitis
Female > Male (2:1)
Finger tumor
Female = Male
Toe tumor

Low Back Pain
Predictors of LBP include poor underlying health, higher weight and body mass index. These associations are stronger in females than males.

Lupus Erythematosus
Female > Male (3:1)
Localized Discoid
Epitheliomas may occasionally appear in healed scars, usually after 20 years of disease and are more common in men.
Female > Male (9:1)
Widespread Discoid
Female > Male (7–10:1)
Systemic
Pregnacy is high risk for both the woman with SLE and the fetus. SLE increases the risk of osteoporosis. The major cause of death in women with SLE is cardiovascular disease, associated with accelerated atherosclerosis. The risk of myocardial infarction is higher in women with SLE compared to normal women.
Women tend to show first symptoms during childbearing years whereas men tend to show disease later in life.

Males have more renal disease (nephropathy and nephrotic syndrome), vascular thrombosis, pleuropericardial disease, peripheral neuropathy and seizures. Males have a higher mortality rate and more severe course than females. Males tend to have more serositis at presentation. Some studies show that males have more discoid lesions but lower incidence of arthritis and malar rash. Males may also have a higher frequency of thrombocytopenia, vasculitis, hemolytic anemia and hepatospenomegaly. In one series males had increased prevalence of anti-dsDNA antibodies compared to women.

Males tend to present more often with serositis.

Men are more likely to have seizures.

Males with SLE have a lower prevalence (32% vs. 43–50%) of 7S IgM and a higher prevalence of IgA deficiency (9.7% vs. 1–4.6%).

Systemic onset in children shows a Female: Male ratio of 4.3:1.

Madelung's Deformity
Female > Male (4:1)

Malignant Fibrous Histiocytoma
Male > Female (3:2)

Meniscal Tear
Male > Female

Metaphyseal Chondrodysplasia, Schmid Type
Males more severely affected.

Metatarsalgia
Female > Male

Microscopic Polyangiitis
Male > Female (1.5:1)

Milwaukee Shoulder
Female > Male

Mixed Connective Tissue Disease
Female > Male (8:1)

Morton Neuroma
   Female > Male (5:1)

Multicentric Reticulohistiocystosis
   Female > Male (2:1)

Myositis Ossificans, Localized
   Male > Female

Myositis Ossificans Progressiva
   Male > Female

Nonarticular Rheumatism of Limbs (Growing Pains)
   Female > Male

Nonossifying Fibroma
   Male > Female

Osgood-Schlatter Disease
   Male > Female (2–3:1)
   The predominant age is 10–16 years in females, 11–18 years in males.

Osteitis Condensans Ilii
   Female > Male

Osteoarthritis
   Female > Male
   Males and females are equally prone to development of osteoarthritis but more joints are affected in females.
   Osteoarthritis related disability is more common in females.
   Osteoarthritis of the hip is slightly more common in males and of the knee in females.

Osteoarthritis of Patellofemoral Joint
   Female > Male

Osteochondritis Dissecans
   Male > Female (3:1)

Osteochondrosis
   Male > Female (3:1)

Osteogenic Sarcoma
   Male > Female (3.7:2.9)
   The knee is the most common site, which peaks in the 2nd decade.

Osteoid Osteoma of the Foot
>   Male > Female

Osteomalacia and Rickets
>   Female > Male (slightly)

Osteomyelitis
>   Male > Female (2.5:1)

Osteonecrosis
>   Male > Female
>   The proximal femur is the most common site and most prevalent in males in the 3rd–6th decade. The distal femur is the second most common site and most common in females in the 6th–7th decade.

Osteoporosis
>   Female > Male (2:1)
>   There is a 30–40% cumulative prevalence in women, a 5–15% cumulative prevalence in men.
>   Osteoporosis related fractures occur in 50% of females and 20% of males > 65 years of age.
>   The cutoff value for osteoporosis at the femoral neck is < 0.56 g/cm^2 in women and < 0.59 g/cm^2 in men.
>   Primary osteoporosis occurs in 80% of women and 60% of men.
>   Secondary osteoporosis occurs in 40% of men and 20% of women.
>   Osteoporotic fracture age-standardized mortality ratio is greater in men.
>> Proximal Femur: women 2.18, men 3.17
>> Vertebra: women 1.92, men 2.38
>> Other major and minor fractures: women 1.92 and 0.75; men 2.22 and 1.45 respectively
>
>   Females tend to have twice as many symptomatic vertebral fractures.
>> 40% of women and 13% of men will experience a hip, vertebral or forearm osteoporotic fracture during their lifetime.
>
>   In young people risk of fracture is higher in males, but after age 45 years, the risk is higher in females.
>   Type 1 osteoporosis primarily affects postmenopausal females (6:1).
>   Type II osteoporosis: Female > Male (2:1)
>   Women are more likely to have severe vertebral fractures and more prominent kyphosis than men.

A maternal history of hip fracture increases the odds ratio of hip fracture in their daughters by 2.0.
Fall frequency is lower in elderly men than elderly women and when they fall women are more likely to land on their hips.

Osteosarcoma
    Male > Female

Pachydermoperiostosis
    Male > Female

Paget's Disease of the Bone
    Male > Female (2:1)

Panner's Disease
    Male > Female

Partial Hypoxanthine Guanine Phosphoribosyltransferase Deficiency
    Male > Female

Patellar Tendinitis
    Male > Female
    Torque production at their knees is greater in males.

Patellofemoral Instability and Misalignment
    Female > Male
    However, the incidence of acute dislocations is higher in men.
    Females have more difficulty with lateral patellar tracking.

Patellofemoral Pain Syndrome
    Female > Male (3:1)

Pellegrinim Steida Syndrome
    Male > Female

Pelvic Insufficiency Fracture
    Female > Male

Peroneal Muscular Atrophy
    Female > Male

Pes Planus
    Female > Male

Piriformis Syndrome
    Female > Male

Plantar Fasciitis
: Female > Male (2:1)

Polyarteritis Nodosa
: Male > Female (2:1)

Polymyalgia Rheumatica
: Female > Male (2:1)
PMR with an erythrocyte sedimentation rate < 40 is seen more in men. Men with PMR tend to be younger and have lower frequency of fever than women.

Polymyositis/Dermatomyositis
: Female > Male (1.7–2:1) overall
The relative risk of cancer in polymyositis is 1.8 in males and 1.7 in females, whereas the relative risk of cancer in dermatomyositis is 2.4 in males and 3.4 in females.

Postenteric Reactive Arthritis
: Male > Female (slightly)
: Shigella: Male > Female (9:1)
: Salmonella: Male > Female (1.6:1)
: Campylobacter: Male > Female (1.3:1)
: Yersinia: Female > Male (1.1:1)
: Sexually-acquired: Male > Female (28:1)

Posterior Tibial Insufficiency
: Female > Male

Posterior Tibial Tendonitis
: Female > Male
Primarily in overweight, elderly females.

Primary Biliary Cirrhosis
: Female > Male (9:1)

Primary Hypertrophic Osteoarthropathy
: Male > Female (9:1)

Primary Vasculitis of the Central Nervous System
: Male > Female

Pronator Syndrome
: Female > Male (4:1)

Psoriatic Arthritis
    Female > Male (slightly)
    Female gender is a risk for more severe disease.
    Males are more likely to develop spondyloarthropathy (occurs in 20–40% of persons with psoriatic arthritis) and tend to have more severe spondyloarthropathy.

Psuedogout
    Female > Male (1.5:1)
    Rarely, mostly elderly females may have destructive lesions of the knees, shoulders and hips.

Pustulosis Palmaris et Plantaris
    Female > Male

Raynaud's Disease
    Female > Male

Raynaud's Phenomenon
    Female > Male (4:1)
            Primary form
    Female = Male
            Secondary form

Reflex Sympathetic Dystrophy
    Female > Male

Reiter's Syndrome
    Male > Female (5:1)
    Whites > Blacks

Relapsing Polychondritis
    Female > Male (3:1)

Remitting Seronegative Symmetrical Synovitis with Pitting Edema
    Male > Female (2:1)

Repetitive Motion Disorders
    Female > Male (3:1)

Retrocalcaneal Bursitis
    Female > Male
    Common in adolescent girls wearing high heels.

Retropatellar Pain
Female > Male

Rhabdomyolysis
Male > Female
Due to a greater incidence of trauma in males.

Rhabdomyosarcoma
Male > Female (slightly)

Rheumatic Fever
The incidence of chorea is equal among prepubescent boys and girls, but this manifestation is absent in the sexually mature male and exaggerated during pregnancy.
There is an increased frequency of tight mitral stenosis in the female and aortic stenosis in the male.

Rheumatoid Arthritis
Female > Male (2–4:1)
Onset in persons > 60 years old is more common in males.
In young adults, females tend to have a worse outcome with more swollen and tender joints and erosions.
Females exhibit greater overall incidence and prevalence of articular involvement but males exhibit more systemic disease.
Men may have higher prevalence of erosive disease but females experience more severe consequences of joint damage.
Even though women have less overall systemic inflammation, they tend to have more destructive changes in the tendons, soft tissue and joint cavity.
Males tend to have more rheumatoid nodules (2:1) and more rheumatoid lung disease (6:1).
Women tend to have more sicca syndrome (3:1).
Life expectancy is decreased 4 years in males and 10 years in females.
Pleural effusions occur more often in men (70–95%).
Males with RA tend to have higher rheumatoid factor titers.

Rheumatoid Arthritis of the Foot
Female > Male (3:1)

Rotator Cuff Syndrome
Male > Female

Rubella Arthralgia
    Female > Male

Sacrococcygeal Teratoma
    Female > Male (3:1)
    Most common fetal neoplasm.

Sarcoidosis
    Female > Male (8:1)
    An acute myopathy with an abnormal EMG is more common in females.
    Black > White

Scaphoid Bone Fracture
    Male > Female

Scheuermann's Disease
    Male > Female

Scleroderma
    Females = Males
        < 8 years of age
    Female > Male (3–4:1)
        > 8 years of age, but up to 15 times greater in females between 15–44 years of age compared to males.
    Scleroderma may be the initial manifestation of a malignacy and females three times more likely to present with signs of scleroderma.

Scoliosis
    Female > Male (7:1)
        Overall
    Female > Male (3–6:1)
        For curves < 10 degrees
    Female > Males (10:1)
        For curves > 30 degrees
    Females progressively curve more.
    In adolescent idiopathic scoliosis, females tend to be more severely affected, but male:female ratio is equal.
    In children 3–10 years of age the male to female ratio is about equal, but in older children Females > Males.
    Adult scoliosis: 80% of cases are females with onset usually at 30–40 years of age.

Septic Arthritis
- Male > Female (2:1)
- Lower extremity accounts for 80% of cases.
- 90% are monoarticular.

Shoulder Injury in Sports
- Female > Male
- Female's shorter upper extremity and body may increase the demand on the shoulder.
- Females are more prone to multidirectional instability.
- Females are more prone to tendonitis of shoulder because the untrained shoulder girdle is weaker in females. This is often seen in throwing and racket sports.

Shoulder Pain
- Female > Male (2.5:1.9)

Sjogren's Syndrome
- Female > Male (9:1)

Sjogren-like Syndrome in AIDS
- Male > Female

Slipped Capital Femoral Epiphysis
- Male > Female (3:2)
- Left hip more often involved than right hip.
- Bilateral disease is more common in blacks.

Slipped Capital Femoral Epiphysis with Chondrolysis
- Female > Male
- Blacks, Hispanics > Whites

Spinal Stenosis, Lumbar
- Male > Female (slightly)

Spondyloepiphyseal Dysplasia Tarda
- Male > Female

Spondylolysis
- Female > Male
- Occurs 4 times as often in female gymnasts.

Sprains and Strains
- Male > Female

Stress Fracture
    Female > Male (up to 12 times greater)
    Femur, pelvic rami and tibial stress fractures are more common in females.

Subcutaneous Achilles Tendonitis
    Female > Male

Syndactyly of Hand
    Male > Female

Synovial Chondroma
    Male > Female (2:1)
    Primarily in middle-aged men. However middle-aged women are more likely to be affected in the temporomandibular joint.

Synovial Plicae, Symptomatic
    Female > Male

Synovial Sarcoma
    Male > Female (slightly)

Synovitis, Pigmented Villonodular
    Male = Female
            Diffuse form
    Female > Male
            Focal form

Synovitis, Transient
    Male > Female (1.5:1)

Takayasu's Arteritis
    Female > Male
    14% of cases are in men.

Tarsal Coalition
    Male > Female

Tarsal Tunnel Syndrome
    Female > Male

Temporomandibular Joint Syndrome
    Female > Male (3:1)

Tendinitis
    Male > Female (slightly)

Thoracic Outlet Syndrome
Female > Male

Thumb Arthritis
Female > Male (10–20:1)
Occurs at the basilar joint of the thumb.

Transient Synovitis of Hip
Male > Female (2–3:1)
More common in whites and < 5% are bilateral.

Trigger Digit
Female > Male (4:1)
In adults, the middle finger most often affected, but in children the thumb most affected.

Trochanteric Bursitis
Female > Male (4:1)

Tuberculous Arthritis
Male > Female

Twelfth Rib Syndrome
Female > Male (3:1)

Urticarial Vasculits
Female > Male

Uveitis in Juvenile Rheumatoid Arthritis
Female > Male

Vertebral Fracture
Lifetime risk is 15.6% in females and 5% in males.

Viral Arthritis
Hepatitis B: Female > Male
Rubella: Female > Male (5:1)
Parvovirus: Female > Male
Mumps: Male > Females
Varicella-Zoster: Female > Male

Weber Christian Disease
Female > Male

Wegener's Granulomatosis
Male > Female (3:2)

Whipple's Disease
  Male > Female

Reproductive Health

Anatomy and Physiology

The pelvic cavity is longer and more conical in males and shorter and more cylindrical in females. The male iliac crest is more rugged and more medially inclined at its anterior end, whereas the female crests are less curved in all parts. Overall pelvic dimensions such as intercristal measurements are greater and markings for muscle attachments and ligaments more pronounced in males. Pelvic type is described as dolichopellic in males and mostly mesatipellic and brachypellic in females. The pelvic outlet anteroposterior diameter is 80 mm in males and 125 mm in females; the transverse diameter is 85 mm in males and 118 mm in females; and the oblique diameter is 100 mm in males and 118 mm in females. The pelvic inlet anteroposterior diameter is 100 mm in males and 112 mm in females; the transverse diameter is 125 mm in males and 131 mm in females; and the oblique diameter is 120 mm in males and 125 mm in females. The pelvic cavity anteroposterior diameter is 105 mm in males and 130 mm in females; the transverse diameter is 120 mm in males and 125 mm in females; and the oblique diameter is 110 mm in males and 131 mm in females. The obturator foramen is larger and more oval shaped in males and more triangular shaped in females. The sacral basal articular facet for the 5th lumbar vertebra and intervening disc is >1/3 of the total sacral basal width in males but < 1/3 in females whose sacrum is relatively broader. The sacral alae is broader in females. The acetabulum is larger in males and its diameter about equal to the distance between its anterior rim and symphysis but in females the acetabular diameter is less than this distance. The female symphysis and adjoining parts of the pubis and ischium are less in height producing a somewhat triangular obturator foramen in females as opposed to an ovoid shape in males. The subpubic arch below the symphysis and between the inferior pubic rami is more angular in males (50–60 degrees) compared to the more rounded shape in females (80–85 degrees). The pubic tubercles are more separated in the female. The ischiopubic rami are lighter and narrower near the symphysis in females. In males they bear a rough, everted area for attachment of the penile crura. Ischial spines are closer in males and are inturned. The greater sciatic notch is usually wider in females. Its width and angle yield mean values of 50.4 degrees and 74.4 degrees for males and females respectively. The greater angle is associated with greater backward sacral tilt and greater anteroposterior pelvic diameter in females. Female sacra are less curved, and the curvature being most prominent between the first and second segments and the third and fifth with an intervening flatter section. Whereas male sacra are more evenly curved, relatively narrow and long and more often exceeding 5 segments. The sacral index (compares sacral breadth with length) is on average 105% in males and 115% in females. Auricular surfaces of the sacrum are relatively smaller and more oblique in females. The dorsal auricular border is more concave in females. The pelvic part of the chilotic line is more predominant in females compared to the sacral part in males. A puboischial index (based on maximum length of the ischium and pubis measured from the acetabular junction) produces values of 83.7% in males and 100% in females. The sacroiliac joint is more curved and irregular in males.

Sex determination and differentiation are sequential processes that involve chromosomal sex in the zygote at the moment of conception, determination of gonadal sex by the genetic sex, determination of phenotypic sex by the gonads. Then, at puberty the development of secondary sexual characteristics provides more visible phenotypic signs of sexual dimorphism. During early development, the gonads of the fetus are undifferentiated. All fetal genitalia are the same and are phenotypically female. After 6–7 weeks of gestation however, the expression of genes on the Y chromosome induces changes that result in the development of the testes. The production of testosterone at about 9 weeks gestation results in the development of the reproductive tract and the masculinization (the normal development of male traits) of the brain and genital tract. The actual dimorphic physical changes of puberty are primarily due to testosterone secretion by the Leydig cells in boys and estrogen secretion by the granulosa cells in girls.

Inhibin B concentrations are elevated in males for the first 2 years of life and increase to adult levels at puberty. In prepubertal females levels are low or undetectable. A sharp increase occurs in females through midpuberty and then a decline occurs.

Leptin levels are higher in females at birth and again in late puberty and adulthood. The levels in boys peak at Tanner stage 2 and decrease by stage 5 whereas in girls the leptin levels increase in breast stage 2 and peak at breast stage 5. The rise in leptin levels occurs 1 year earlier in girls.

Nonpregnant females have higher concentrations of human choriogonadotropin in serum and urine than men. The average weight of the male newborn is 200 grams more than the female newborn.

Homologies Between Female and Male Sexual Structures

Primordial Structure	*Male Derivative*	*Female Derivative*
GONAD		
Indifferent gonad derived from:		
Coelomic epithelium	Semineferous tubules	Graafian follicles
Mesenchymal cell mass	Sertoli cells	Granulosa cells
Mesonephric elements	Leydig cells	Theca cells
		Interstitial cells
	Rete testes	Rete ovarii
	Septa and tunica albuginea	
	Tunica vaginalis	
	Spermatogonia ——> sperm	
GENITAL DUCTS		
Mesonephric tubules	Ductuli efferentes	Epoophoron
	Aberrant ductules	Paroophoron
Mesonephric (wolffian) ducts	Epididymis	Gartner duct
	Vas deferens	
	Seminal Vesicles	
	Ejaculatory ducts	
	Appendix testis (hydatid)	
EXTERNAL GENITALIA		
Genital tubercle	Penis	Clitoris
	Corpora cavernosa	Corpora cavernosa
	Glans penis	Glan clitoris

Urethral folds	Corpus spongiosum	Labia minora
Labioscrotal swellings	Scrotum & ventral epidermis of penis	Labia majora Paraurethral glands
Urogenital sinus	Prostate	Bartholin glands
	Bulbourethral glands	Lower vagina
	Prostatic utricle	

Anatomic and Physiologic Alterations Occurring During Pregnancy

SYSTEM	CHANGE
Cardiovascular	Cardiac output increased by 50%
	Plasma volume increased by 50%
	Peripheral vascular resistance decreased
	Vena caval compression
Gastrointestinal	Decreased motility
	Decreased gastrointestinal sphincter competency
	Intra-abdominal organ displacement
Genitourinary	Enlarged ovarian venous plexus
	Dilatation of renal system
Laboratory Data	Increased WBC count
	Decreased hematocrit level
	Increased fibrinogen and factor VIII levels
Respiratory	Decreased residual lung volume
	Decreased Pao_2
	Chronic respiratory alkalosis

Diseases

Breast Abscess
   Female > Male

Breast Cancer
   Female > Male (99:1)
   One in eight females will develop breast cancer in their lifetime.
   77% of breast cancers occur in women > age 50 years.
   Average age at diagnosis is 10 years older in males and involves the pectoralis major muscle more commonly in males.
   Males present with more advanced disease.
   Male breast cancer is more likely to be estrogen receptor positive (84%) than female breast cancer (57%).

Breast cancer susceptibility genes include BRCA1 and BRCA2. About 1 in 400 females will carry a germ line mutation for BRCA1. Male BRCA2 carriers have a higher risk for breast cancer.

The incidence of breast cancer in men has remained stable in contrast to the increasing incidence in women over the last 40 years.

The median age at diagnosis is 68 years in men versus 63 years in women. The bimodal age distribution seen in women is absent in men.

Breast cancer in men may be a marker for Klinefelter syndrome; between 4–20% of men with breast cancer have been found to have the syndrome.

BRCA1 and BRCA2 breast cancer susceptibility genes are thought to account for most hereditary breast cancers in women, but only BRCA2 mutations in men predispose to breast cancer.

In men, almost all of the noninvasive cancers are ductal carcinoma in situ.

Lobular cancer in situ is rare in men, because of the absence of terminal lobules in the normal male breast. Ductal carcinoma in situ of the male breast is almost always low to intermediate grade, and 75% of cases are a papillary subtype which is different from that of the female breast.

Lobular carcinoma is much less common in men than in women.

The rarer subtypes such as medullary, tubular, mucinous, and squamous carcinomas are slightly more uncommon in men than in women.

Carcinomas of the male breast have a higher rate of hormone receptor positivity than do carcinomas of the female breast. Men, in contrast to women, do not have a higher incidence of estrogen receptor-positive tumors with advancing age.

Men have higher rates of expression of the molecular marker Bcl-2 than women.

Chancroid
Male > Female (10:1)
It seems the environment provided by the foreskin makes men more susceptible to the bacteria responsible for chancroid.

Chlamydia
Female > Male (6–7:1)
The rate is 350 per 100,000 females and 60 per 100,000 men.

Younger females more susceptible to gonorrhea and chlamydial associated infection than older females.

Women are more likely to develop pelvic inflammatory disease (PID) than men to develop epididymo-orchitis.

Congenital Anomalies of Genital Organs
Male > Female (13:1)

Cystosarcoma Phyllodes
Female only

Delayed Puberty
Male > Female

Dyspareunia
Female > Male
About 15% of adult females will have dyspareunia on a few occasions during a year. About 1–2% will have painful intercourse more frequently.

Fibroadenoma of Breast
Female > Male

Fibrocystic Breast Disease
Female > Male (almost all cases in females)

Galactorrhea
Female > Male
Males rarely affected.

Genital Herpes
Female > Male
Males more likely to be asymptomatic with newly acquired infection. Annual risk of susceptible female acquiring disease from an infected male is 10–30%: for susceptible male from infected female is 5%.

Gonorrhea
Male > Female
About 30 years ago, the ratio was 4:1 but is now getting closer to 1:1.
In females, salpingitis is common. In men, epididymitis may occur. A single episode of intercourse with an infected partner carries a transmission risk of 20–25% for males; female partners of infected males have a 50–80% risk of infection.

Of infected females, 30–60% will be asymptomatic or minimally affected as will up to 40% of males.
Disseminated gonococcal infections occur mainly in females.

Herpes Simplex Type 2
   Female > Male (1.4:1)
   Seroprevalence surveys find antibody in 26% of females and 18% of men.
   Transmission of herpes from infected male to uninfected female is greater (annual risk of 15–30%) than from infected female to uninfected male (4–6% annual risk).
   Females have more painful recurrences.
   About 50% of males have recurrence within 4 months whereas 50% of females will not have recurrence until 8 months after initial outbreak.

HIV
   Males > Females
   Females are more likely to be infected with multiple strains all at once, compared to men that are usually infected with only one strain. Levels of HIV-1 RNA may be lower in women than men at the same CD4 count, but women have higher CD4 counts at the time of AIDS diagnosis.
   The rate of HIV infection is increasing faster in women, who accounted for 30% of cases in 1999 in the United States.
   Use of antiretroviral therapy has been associated with abnormal accumulations of body fat and elevated cholesterol, triglyceride and glucose levels with development of insulin resistance and is termed lipodystrophy syndrome. Women with this syndrome are more likely than men to have increases in abdominal fat (93% vs. 76%), and breast size (74% vs. 31%) whereas men are more likely to have lipoatrophy in the limbs (69% vs. 53%) and buttocks (60% vs. 45%). Men are more likely to develop high triglyceride (63% vs. 26%) and cholesterol (50% vs. 26%) levels. However women have a higher risk for adverse drug effects (37% vs. 25%).

Infertility
   Males are the cause in 20–40%, Females 60–80%

Juvenile Fibroadenoma of Breast
   Female > Male

Lymphogranuloma Venereum
    Male > Female (5:1)
    The genital (inguinal) syndrome occurs more in males, but acute rectal syndrome occurs more in females.

Mammary Duct Ectasia
    Female > Male

Mastalgia
    Female > Male

Mucocutaneous Candidiasis
    Female > Male

Nongonoccocal Urethritis
    Male > Female
    Asymptomatic infection occurs in 28% of contacts of women with chlamydial cervical infection.
    NGU has a greater morbidity than gonococcal urethritis.

Papillomatosis of Breast
    Female > Male

Precocious Puberty
    Female > Male
        Idiopathic form
    In males, precocious puberty is usually due to a teratoma of the pineal gland, whereas in females it is usually caused by an estrogen secreting tumor or hypothalmic hamartoma.

Sexual Aversion Disorder
    Female > Male
    Is accompanied by reactions of anxiety and disgust.

Sexual Dysfunction
    Female > Male (4:3)
    Lack of interest is most common problem in women; premature climaxing is the number one problem in men. Erectile dysfunction occurs in 35% of men age 40–70 years. Anorgasmia is more common in females. 20–30% of females have difficulty achieving orgasms.
    1/3rd of women and 1/6th of men are uninterested in sex.
    1/5th of women in one study said that sex provided little pleasure compared to 1/10th of men.

Men in poor health are at risk for sexual dysfunction, especially erectile failure.

Early depression is associated with hypoactive sexual desire in women.

Women in poor health are at risk for sexual pain disorders.

Past history of sexually transmitted disease increases the odds of low desire in women but not men.

Sexual abuse is a significant risk for desire and arousal disorders in women more than men.

Sexual Pain Disorder
Female > Male
It occurs in 10–15% of women.

Sexually Transmitted Disease
Women suffer more frequently from chronic pelvic pain and infertility than men after an STD.

The rate of epididymo-orchitis is 1/2 to 2/3rds the rate of PID in females.

Some studies show the rate of transmission from chlamydia and gonorrhea and HIV are more likely to occur from males to females than from females to males.

Syphilis
Male > Female (1.5:1)
Syphilis has been increasing in males since the early 1990's.

The median duration of the primary and secondary stages in males is 3.1 months and in females 4.4 months.

The median duration of the secondary stage alone is 2.1 months in males and 3.5 months in females.

In males, the lesions feel firm and rubbery, whereas in females the lesions are characterized by edematous induration.

Before antibiotics, cardiovascular involvement was noted in 13.6% of males and 7.6% of females with syphilis. Neurosyphilis developed in 9.4% of males and 5% of females before antibiotics were introduced.

Dementia paralytica developed in 2.5% of males and 1.4% of females prior to effective antibiotic therapy.

Interstitial keratitis developed at an average age of 13.5 years in males and 27.1 years in females with congenital syphilis.

Testicle Cancer
    Male only
    White > Black (4:1)

Trichomoniasis
    Female > Male
    Both sexes affected but women are more symptomatic (75% vs. 10%).
    Makes up 10–25% of vaginal infections.

Uterine Fibroids
    Females only
    Black >White
    ~ 50% of Black Females >30 years old are affected.
    ~ 20% of White Females >30 years are affected.

Infectious Diseases

Anatomy and Physiology

Adaptive immunity markedly varies by sex, innate immunity varies less. Females tend to have a more aggressive immune response to infectious challenges. Gonadal hormones affect immune and inflammatory cell responses but men and women respond in a similar manner to infection. Estrogens upregulate and androgens downregulate the cellular effectors of adaptive immunity: lympocytes, macrophages, and dendritic cells. The adaptive immune response varies during the menstrual cycle. Studies in posttraumatic morbidity patients suggest that females are immunologically better positioned toward a septic challenge.

Vaccination:
    Vaccination induces higher antibody levels in females.
    Adverse systemic reactions to immunization, especially arthritis, are more common in females.
    Hepatitis A: Antibody titers are higher in females after immunization.
    Hepatitis B: Antibody titers are higher in females after immunization.
    Influenza: More local and systemic adverse effects in females after vaccination.
    Rubella: Arthritis is 3.5 times more common in girls after vaccination.
    Measles: Antibody-dependent cell cytotoxicity is lower in females but neutralizing antibody levels are equal in the sexes.

Diseases

Actinomycosis
    Male > Female (2–3:1)

Amebiasis
    Male ≥ Female
    Male are more likely to develop liver abscess.
    Males have greater occupational exposure.

Amebic Liver Abscess
    Male > Female (10–15:1)

Anal and Rectal Abscess
    Male > Female (2.5:1)

Anthropophilic Dermatophytosis
    Male > Female

Arenavirus Infection, South American
    Male > Female

Arthritis, Bacterial
    Female > Male (4:1)
        Neisserial
        Arthritis occurs in 0.6% of the 3% of females with gonorrhea.
        Arthritis occurs in 0.1% of the 0.7% of men with gonorrhea.
    Male > Female (2:1)
        Non-Neisserial
    Male = Female
        Subacute bacterial endocarditis-related

Arthritis, Infectious Granulomatous
    Male > Female
        Brucella and Mycobacteria
    Female > Male
        Fungal

Ascariasis
    Female > Male (slightly)

Aspergillosis
    Male > Female

Babesiosis
    Male > Female

Bartonella Infection
    Male > Female
    Nonbacilliformis Bartonellosis infection

Blastomycosis
    Male > Female (9:1)
    Although in outbreaks, the sex ratio shows no difference.

Botulism
    Male = Female
            Foodborne and Infantile
    Male > Female
            Wound

Brain Abscess
    Male > Female (2:1)

Breast Abscess
    Female > Male

Brucellosis
    Male > Female
            Occupational exposure
    Female ≥ Male
            Milk exposure
    Spondylitis due to Brucella is more common in males (7:3) than females.

California Encephalitis
    Male > Female (2:1)

Campylobacter Jejuni Infection
    Male > Female

Capillariasis
    Male > Female

Chagas Disease
: Female > Male (5.6:4.4)
  There is a 5% chance of congenital transmission.

Chancroid
: Male > Female

Chlamydia Pneumoniae Infection
: Male > Female

Chromoblastomycosis
: Male > Female

Chromomycosis
: Male > Female

Chronic Oral Atrophic Candidiasis
: Female > Male

Coccidioidomycosis
: Male > Female
    For dissemination of infection.
  Pregnant females are at greater risk.
  Males have worse prognosis.
  Females more likely to have erythema nodusum (better prognosis).

Colorado Tick Fever
: Male > Female (2:1)

Community-Acquired Pneumonia
: Male sex is a risk factor for mortality.

Croup
: Male > Female (3:2)

Cryptococcosis
: Male > Female (2:1)
  Reflects HIV prevalence.

Cytomegalovirus Inclusion Disease
: Male > Female
  Probably reflects HIV prevalence in homosexual males.

Endocardial Abscess in Children
: Male > Female
  Majority occur in males.

Epstein-Barr Virus Infection
   Male = Female
   Peak incidence is about 2 years earlier in females.
   Splenic rupture more in males.

Erhlichiosis
   Male > Female (3:1)

Filariasis
   Male > Female
   There is a higher prevalence of hydrocoele in men as compared to lymphedema in women in the genital region.
   Age at onset appears higher in women.

Giardiasis
   Male > Female (slightly)

Gingivitis
   Male > Female

Gonorrhea
   Male > Female
      Adults
      Males are more symptomatic.
   Female > Male
      Children and adolescents

Granuloma Inguinale
   Male > Female

Hepatitis A
   Male > Female (slightly)

Hepatitis B
   The rate of hepatitis B in adults is greater in males but in adolescents the rate is higher in females.

Hepatitis B, Fulminant
   Male > Female (2:1)

Hepatitis C
   Male > Female (2:1)

Hepatitis E
    Male > Female
    Pregnant females are at risk of severe illness.

Herpes, Genital
    Female > Male

Histoplasmosis
    Male = Female
        Acute
    Male > Female
        Chronic pulmonary histoplasmosis
        Usually occurs in white males with history of obstructive lung disease.
    Female > Male (5:1)
        Disseminated

Histoplasmosis Capsulatum
    Female = Male
    Clinical disease is more common in males (4:1), but women are more likely to have arthralgias, myalgias and skin manisfestations. Chronic pulmonary form is more common in males.

Histoplasmosis Duboisii
    Male > Female

Human Granulocytic Erlichiosis
    Male > Female (3:1)

Human Immunodeficiency Virus Infection
    Male > Female (3:1)
        Adults, but rate is increasing in females.
    Male = Female
        Children
    Females have increased risk for candida esophagitis and bacterial pneumonia while men have higher risk of Kaposi's sarcoma and oral hairy leukoplakia.
    Although the initial HIV-1 RNA load is lower in women, the rate to progression to AIDS is similar to males.
    Females have more rapid decline in CD4+ cell counts over time than males.

Females may achieve virologic suppression at a faster rate and have a more durable response than men after antiviral medication.

Infection After Trauma
>   Male > Female (1.5:1)
>   There is an increased risk of infection after trauma in males.
>   Male gender is a risk factor for pneumonia, pelvic and abdominal abscess, meningitis, and wound infections requiring operative debridement after major trauma.

Infection in Hospitalized Persons
>   Male gender is a risk factor for the development of nosocomial bloodstream infections.
>   Female gender is a predictor of mortality in Enterococcal bacteremia. Females may have a higher mortality rate from lung and necrotizing soft tissue infections.

Infective Endocarditis
>   Male > Female (slightly)

Invasive Mycotic Infections
>   Male > Female (2.8:1)
>   The ratio decreases to 1.3:1 (male to female) if HIV patients are excluded.

Kawasaki Syndrome
>   Male > Female (1.6:1)

Kuru
>   Female > Male
>   Only females eat the infected brain tissue for cultural reasons.

Lacrosse Encephalitis
>   Male > Female (2:1)

Legionnaire's Disease
>   Male > Female (3:1)

Leishmaniasis
>   Male > Female

Lemierre's Syndrome
>   Male > Female (3:1)

Leprosy
> Male > Female (overall)
>> Especially the lepromatous form.
> Male = Female
>> Childhood
> Male > Female (2:1)
>> Adult
> 94% of antineutrophil cytoplasmic antibody-positive patients are males.
> Longer delay in identifying skin changes in females.

Leptospirosis
> Male > Female (4:1)

Listeriosis
> Male > Female
> Pregnant women are more likely to get listeriosis (up to 20 times).

Lung Abscess
> Male > Female (4:1)

Lyme Disease
> Male > Female (1–2:1)

Lymphogranuloma Venereum
> Male > Female (5:1)

Measles
> Females have more arthralgias.
> Girls have higher case fatality rates (because of lack of immunization).

Meningococcal Meningitis
> Male > Female

Microsporium Tinea Capitis
> Male > Female

Molluscum Contagiosum
> Male > Female

Mucocutaneous Candidiasis
> Female > Male

Mumps
   Male > Female (2.3:1.7)

Mycobacterium Avium, Nodular Form
   Female > Male
   There is an increasing incidence in middle-aged females without underlying lung disease or immune deficiency.
   Females predominate in people without predisposing risk factors.

Mycobacterium Chelonei
   Female > Male

Mycobacterium Fortuitum
   Male > Female

Mycobacterium Haemophilum
   Male > Female (2:1)

Mycobacterium Kansasii
   Male > Female (3:1)
   Musculoskeletal infections due to M. Kansasii are twice as common in males.

Mycobacterium Marinum
   Male > Female

Mycobacterium Terrae
   Male > Female (3:2)

Mycobacterum Tuberculosis
   Male > Female (1.5–2:1)
   However females have a higher progression from infection to disease and a higher case fatality rate.
   More males have a positive tuberculin skin test; this may reflect higher infection rate in men or altered immune response in females.

Neonatal Meningitis
   Male > Female

Neonatal Sepsis
   Male > Female (2:1)

Nocardiosis
   Male > Female (3:1)

Infectious Diseases

Nosocomial Blood Infections
Male > Female
Male gender is a risk factor for nosocomial blood stream infections. However, female gender is a predictor for mortality in patients with Enterococcus bloodstream infections.
Women may have a higher mortality among patients with necrotizing soft tissue infection, nosocomial pneumonia, and a higher rate of multisystem organ dysfunction in postop cardiac patients developing nosocomial infections.

Onchocerciasis
Women report more itching than men.

Osteomyelitis
Male > Female

Otitis Media
Male > Female

Paracoccidioidomycosis
Male > Female (38:1)
It is thought that this large difference is due to the inhibition of hyphae to undergo yeast transformation by estrogen.

Paronychia
Female > Male (3:1)

Parvovirus B19 infection
Female > Male
Adults

Pediculosis
Female > Male

Perianal Cellulitis
Male > Female

Pericarditis
Male > Female (slightly)

Peritonitis, Acute
Male > Female

Pertussis
Female > Male

Pinworms
> Female > Male

Plague
> Male > Female (in U.S)
> Except for the youngest and oldest cases are more likely female.

Pneumocystis Carinii
> Male > Female

Pneumonia, Bacterial
> Male > Female (2:1)

Pneumonia, Mycoplasma
> Male > Female

Post-Surgical Infections
> Male > Female (1.5:1)
> Females are at increased risk (2X) of death from nosocomial pneumonia although pneumonia is more common in men postop. Females with pneumonia have a higher white cell count and a slightly lower body temperature at time of diagnosis than do men. Men are more likely to have pneumonia and bloodstream infections. Females are more likely to have urinary tract infections.

Posttraumatic Sepsis
> Males > Females
> In severely injured patients, sepsis occurred in more males (31% vs. 17%) and multiple organ dysfunction syndrome occurred in more males (30% vs. 16%).
> Plasma levels of procalcitonin and interleukin-6, cytokines and estradiol levels were increased in men in the early posttraumatic event. These changes were not seen in females.

Powassan Encephalitis
> Male > Female (2:1)

Puumala Virus Infection
> Male > Female (2–3:1)
> Causes nephropathic epidemica.

Pyogenic Liver Abscess
> Male > Female (1–2.4:1)

Q-Fever
>   Male > Female (3:1)

Rabies
>   Male > Female (3:1)

Respiratory Syncytial Virus Infection
>   Male = Female
>   >   Outpatient
>
>   Male > Female (1.5:1)
>   >   Hospitalized

Rocky Mountain Spotted Fever
>   Male > Female
>   Due to greater male outdoor activity.

Rubella
>   Male > Female
>   There is a lower immunization rate in boys.
>   Adult females are more likely to have arthritis complications.
>   Males and females have differences in antibody classes during acute infection. IgA anti-E2 antibodies are seen in females but not males. Also lower levels of IgG against structural proteins t E2 are observed in males. Males have earlier onset of E1-specific IgG and IgM antibodies with a higher proportion of total rubella virus antibody response directed to E1 (IgG) of E1 peptide (IgM).

Salmonella Aortitis
>   Male > Female (3:1)

Salmonella Pyomyositis
>   Male > Female (3:1)

Schistosomiasis
>   Males > Females
>   However societal roles and religious practices are important in determining susceptibility to infection.
>   Infection appears to affect the genital tract of females.

Schistosomiasis Haematobia
>   The specific IgA response and production of TGF-beta and Il10 are higher in females.

Schistosoma Mansoni
> Males have an increased risk of severe disease and increased risk of growth deficits compared to females.

Shigellosis
> Female > Male
> Rate is almost twice higher in female adolescents and adults in the US.
> Male homosexuals are at increased risk.

Snowshoe Encephalitis
> Male > Female (5:1)

Sporotrichosis
> Male > Female
> Pulmonary sporotrichosis is usually due to occupational exposure.

Streptococcal Toxic Shock Syndrome
> Male > Female
> No gender preference in Staphylococcal TSS.

Subacute Sclerosing Panencephalitis
> Male > Female
> Occurs in 6–22 per million cases of measles infection.
> Onset is usually before age 20 years.

Syphilis
> Male > Female (1.5:1.1)
>> Adults
>
> Female > Male (2:1)
>> Adolescents

Tick Paralysis
> Female > Male
> Long hair may cause tick to be unnoticed.

Tinea Barbae
> Males only by definition

Tinea Cruris
> Male > Female

Tinea Favosa
> Male = Female

However, chronic infections that extend into adulthood are more common in females.

Tinea Pedis
    Male > Female

Tinea Unguium
    Male > Female

Toxic Shock Syndrome
    Female > Male (3:2)

Trichomoniasis
    Female > Male

Trichophyton Tinea Capitis
    Female > Male

Tuberculosis
    Male > Female
        In older people
    Disease rates are higher in males; young women progress from infection to disease more frequently.
    Females are less compliant with therapy.

Tularemia
    Male > Female
    Especially in rural areas due to occupation and recreation.

Western Equine Encephalitis
    Male > Female (2:1)

Ophthalmology

Anatomy and Physiology

Aging affects the retrobulbar circulation differently by gender. In healthy elderly males, the posterior ciliary arteries' flow velocities and the Pourcelot resistance index are independent of age. But in females end-diastolic velocity decreases with age in both the temporal and nasal posterior ciliary vessel, the peak systolic velocity is constant, and the Pourcelot resistance index in each ciliary artery rises with advancing age.

Increased corneal, lid, and conjunctival edema occurs during certain phases of the menstrual cycle and may alter visual performance. This may complicate fitting of contact lens in women. Corneal thickness also increases with rising progesterone levels during pregnancy. The conjunctiva is an estrogen sensitive epithelial tissue and some studies find that cyclic variation in the maturation index of the cornea parallels the menstrual cycle. Other visual changes noted across the menstrual cycle include color vision, contrast sensitivity, visual fields and visual detection.

Females tend to have higher intraocular pressure than males, especially after age 40 years. The optic disc area is greater in males than in females. Females have greater amounts of lactoferrin and specific tear proteins in their tears than men. Male neonates appear to have a more advanced stage of iris development than female neonates.

The corneas of older men are flatter than older women. The vertical corneal meridian, but not the horizontal, shows gender related changes with ageing. Elderly men have a higher potential for against-the-rule astigmatism.

Females have shorter visual evoked potential latencies for two sized check stimuli subtending 15' and 31'.

Diseases

Abetalipoproteinemia
    Female > Male

Acute Posterior Multifocal Placoid Pigment Epitheliopathy
    Female > Male
    Patient often has upper respiratory infection 1–2 weeks earlier.

Adenocarcinoma of the Lacrimal Gland
    Male > Female (3:1)

Adult Chronic Dacryocystitis
    Female > Male

Alcardi Syndrome
    Female > Male
    X-linked Dominant

Angle Closure Glaucoma
    Female > Male (3:1)
        Whites
    Female = Male
        Blacks

Anterior Uveitis, Acute
    Male > Female

Asteroid Hyalosis
    Male > Female

Atopic Keratoconjunctivitis
    Male > Female

Benign Mixed Tumor of the Lacrimal Gland
    Male > Female (2:1)

Bloch-Sulzberger Syndrome
    Female only
    Lethal in male embryos.

Blue Rod Monochromatism
    Male > Female

Carotid Artery-Cavernous Sinus Fistula
   Female > Male

Cataracts
   Female > Male
   Incidence rises more sharply in ageing women than ageing men. Nuclear and cortical cataracts are associated with elevated cholesterol levels in women but only nuclear cataracts associated with high cholesterol levels in men.
   Nuclear cataracts seem to occur more often in women.

Central Serous Retinopathy
   Male > Female

Chondrodysplasia Punctata, X-Linked Form
   Females only
   Lethal in male embryos.

Choroidal Osteoma
   Female > Male

Choroidemia
   Male > Female
   Female carriers usually show mild abnormalities of the retinal pigment epithelium.

Chronic Cicatricial Conjunctivitis
   Male > Female
   Primarily in patients over age 60 years.

Coats Disease
   Male > Female
   Primarily in males between 18 months–18 years old.

Color Blindness
   Male > Female

Congenital Retinoschisis
   Male > Female

Conjunctival Intraepithelial Epithelioma
   Male > Female

Convergence Insufficiency
   Female > Male

Cranial Arteritis
    Female > Male

Diabetes Mellitus
    Risk of blindness: Nonwhite Female > White Male, Female > Black Male.
    Severe proliferative retinopathy develops more frequently in young men, and blindness is more common in men than women before age 45 years.

Diabetic Retinopathy
    Male = Female
            Juvenile onset
    Female > Male
            Noninsulin dependent diabetes mellitus

Dry Eye Syndrome
    Female > Male
    Primarily in postmenopausal females, and hormone replacement therapy may help these women.

Duane Retraction Syndrome
    Female > Male (5.4:4.6)

Eales Disease
    Male > Female

Episcleritis
    Female > Male (3:1)

Essential Iris Atrophy
    Female > Male

Fabry Disease
    Male > Female

Floppy Eyelids
    Male > Female
    Often have sleep apnea.

Fungal Keratitis
    Male > Female
    Except candida, where 55% are females with debilitating disease. Males usually present with eye trauma.

Glaucoma, Childhood
  Male > Female (2:1)

Gorlin-Goltz Syndrome
  Female > Male (7:1)

Gyrate Atrophy
  Male > Female

Hunter Syndrome II
  Male > Female

Idiopathic Orbital Inflammation (Pseudotumor)
  Male > Female

Incontinentia Pigmenti
  Female only
  Most males die as embryos.

Infraclinoid Aneurysm
  Female > Male

Iridocorneal Endothelial Syndrome
  Female > Male

Keratoconus
  Female > Male (slightly)

Keratomalacia
  Bitot spots are seen especially in boys.

Lacrimal Disorders
  Female > Male (2.5:1)

Laurence-Moon-Biedl-Bardet Syndrome
  Male > Female

Leber's Hereditary Optic Neuropathy
  Male > Female (9:1)

Lowe Syndrome
  Male > Female

Lymphangioma of the Orbit
  Female > Male (3:1)

Macular Degeneration, Age-Related
    Female > Male (1.15:1)
    Over 75 years of age, 1/3 of females have senile macular degeneration, and are twice as likely to have ARMD as men. Females also have higher incidence of exudative macular degeneration.

Malignant Melanoma of the Choroid
    Female > Male (slightly)

Medullated Nerve Fibers
    Male > Female

Metastasis to the Choroid
    Female—breast, lung cancer
    Male—lung, kidney, testicle, prostate cancer

Morning Glory Anomaly of the Optic Disk
    Female > Male (2:1)

Narrow Angle Glaucoma
    Female > Male

Normal Tension Glaucoma
    Female > Male

Ocular Abrasion
    Male > Female

Ocular Albinism
    Male > Female

Ocular Chemical Burn
    Male > Female

Ocular Foreign Body
    Male > Female (slightly)

Ocular Trauma
    Male > Female (3.5:1)

Oculocerebrorenal Syndrome of Lowe
    X-linked males are born with small opacified crystalline lens.
    Female carriers may develop cataracts before age 40 years.

Open Angle Glaucoma
    Male > Female

Before age 50 years.
  Male = Female
    After age 50 years.

Optic Atrophy
  Male > Female
    Inherited Form
  Male > Female
    Head injury

Optic Atrophy, Inherited
  Male > Female

Optic Nerve Sheath Meningioma
  Female > Male (5:1)

Optic Neuritis
  Female > Male

Phyctenular Conjunctivitis
  Female > Male (2:1)

Pigment Dispersion Syndrome
  Male > Female
  Primarily in young men with myopia.

Pituitary Adenoma
  Visual field defects more common in men.

Posterior Vitreous Detachment
  Female > Male

Primary Angle Closure Glaucoma
  Female > Male

Primary Congenital Open-Angle Glaucoma
  Male > Female

Primary Developmental Glaucoma
  Female > Male

Pseudomonas Keratitis
  Male > Female

Pseudotumor Cerebri
   Female > Male
   Primarily obese females of reproductive age.

Reading Problems
   Male > Female
   Schools identify four times as many boys as girls, although epidemiologic studies find that as many girls as boys manifest dyslexia.

Red-Green Color Vision Deficit
   Male > Female (16:1)

Retinal Cavernous Hemangiomatosis
   Female > Male

Retinal Detachment
   Male > Female (3:2)

Retinitis Pigmentosa
   Male > Female (2–3:1)

Retinoschisis, Degenerative
   Female > Male

Retinoschisis, Juvenile X-chromosome Linked
   Male > Female

Retraction Syndrome of Stilling, Turk and Duane
   Female > Male (3:2)
   Left eye affected 75% of the time.

Scleritis
   Female > Male (3:2)

Senile Macular Degeneration
   Female > Male (2:1)
      After age 75 years
   Females also have a higher incidence of exudative macular degeneration.

Superior Limbic Keratoconjunctivitis
   Female > Male

Syphilitic Interstitial Keratitis
   Male > Female

Thyroid Eye Disease
   Female > Male (3:1)

Tonic Pupil
   Female > Male

Trisomy 18 Syndrome
   Female > Male (3:1)

Uveitis
   Male = Female
      Overall
   Male > Female (2.5:1)
      For HLA-B27 anterior uveitis

Vernal Conjunctivitis
   Male > Female (2:1)
      Overall
   Male > Female
      Before puberty
   Male = Female
      After puberty

Vernal Keratoconjunctivitis
   Male > Female

Wildervanck Syndrome
   Female > Male
   Tends to be lethal to male embryos.

X-linked Congenital Cataract
   Male > Female

X-Linked Disorders for Which Phenotypic Evidence of the Carrier State may be Present in Females
   Choroideremia
   Ocular Albinism
   Retinitis Pigmentosa
   Nance-Horan Syndrome
   Blue Cone Monochromatism
   Cone Dystrophy
   X-linked Recessive Congenital Cataracts
   Lowe Syndrome

X-linked Retinoschisis
    Male > Female
    Female may show peripheral retinal alterations.

Otolaryngology

Anatomy and Physiology

The male has a larger pharynx than the female. The pharynx in men is 3.63 ± 0.10 cm² versus 3.20 ± 0.09 cm² in women. Males have a larger change in pharyngeal area with changing lung volume than women (0.60 ± 0.14 cm² versus 0.12 ± 0.12 cm²). In older men, elongation of the laryngeal ventricle is common.

Vocal cords: Prepubertal length: 12–15 mm in boys and girls. Length in adult men is 18–23 mm, compared to 13–18 mm in women.

During puberty the male larynx, cricothyroid cartilage and laryngeal muscles enlarge and the adult male voice is achieved by about age 15 years of age.

The level of androgen and progesterone receptors present in vocal cords are greater in males which may explain why men have deeper voices than women and why women treated with testosterone may develop a deep voice.

Acoustic characteristics of children's speech and voices can identify a child's sex. Vowel formant frequencies differentiate children's sex by 4 years of age while formant frequencies and fundamental frequency differentiate sex after 12 years of age.

Intentional speech: girls generally surpass boys in learning speech sounds and girls tend to be accelerated in articulation skills from about 4 ½ years on. Females normally approximate mature articulation by age 7 years, whereas boys are usually age 8 years old when they reach the same degree of proficiency.

Thyroid Cartilage: In males, the alae of the thyroid cartilage fuse at about 90 degrees making a laryngeal prominence (Adam's apple). In the female, the prominence is absent because of the more oblique fusion angle of 120 degrees. The midline vertical distance from the thyroid notch to inferior border of the thyroid cartilage is about 20 mm in males and 15.5 mm in females. The thyroid cartilage undergoes ossification in the male at about age 20 years of age and a few years later in females.

The cochlea is 13% longer in males than females (37.1 ± 1.6 mm vs. 32.3 ± 1.8 mm). Female newborns' hearing is more sensitive than male newborns and the differences between sexes increases as the frequency increases. Hearing sensitivity and prevalence of spontaneous otoacoustic emissions show gender differences. Spontaneous otoacoustic emissions are more common in females. Auditory brain stem response shows differences in wave V latency between head-sized matched males and females.

In sebum ear wax, the straight odd chain fatty acids show a similar positive correlation with testosterone levels to that of the straight even chain fatty acids in males; while in females, there is no correlation between the amounts of fatty acids and testosterone levels.

Females rate the taste of 6-n-propylthiouracil as more bitter than do males.

Diseases

Acoustic Neuroma
    Female > Male (slightly)

Age-Related Hearing Loss
    Male > Female

Angiofibroma of the Nasopharynx
    Male > Female

Angioleiomyoma of the Larynx
    Male > Female
    Described primarily in elderly men.

Aryepiglottic Zone Carcinoma
    Male > Female (5:1)

Aural Atresia
    Male > Female
    Usually more often involves the right ear.

Autoimmune Inner Ear Disease
    Female > Male (2:1)

Basaloid Squamous Cell Cancer
    Male > Female

Benign Lymphoepithelial Lesion (Mikuliez's Disease)
    Female > Male (4:1)

Brachial Sinus and Fistula
    Female > Male (slightly)

Buccal Cavity and Pharyngeal Cancer
    Male > Female (2:1)

Burning Mouth Syndrome
    Female > Male (5.5:1.6)

Carcinoid of the Larynx
    Male > Female

Carcinoma of the Ear
    Male > Female (4:1)

Cavernous Hemangioma of the Larynx
    Male > Female (2:1)

Choanal Atresia
    Female > Male

Chondrosarcoma of the Larynx
    Male > Female (4:1)

Cicatricial Pemphigoid
    Female > Male (2:1)

Cleft Lip and Palate
    This occurs on the left side more in males than in females.
    Cleft palate is more associated with olfactory deficits in boys than girls.

Congenital Epulis
    Female > Male

Conversion Reaction Dysphonia
    Female > Male

Cystic Adenoid Cancer (Brooke's Tumor)
    Female > Male

Extramedullary Plasmacytoma
    Male > Female

Extramedullary Plasmacytoma of the Larynx
    Male > Female

Fibrosarcoma of the Larynx
    Male > Female (4:1)

Fibrous Dysplasia
    Female > Male
    Primarily affects maxilla.

Follicular Carcinoma of the Thyroid
    Female > Male (3:1)

Functional Pitch Disorder
    Male > Female

Glomus Jugulare Tumor
    Female > Male (5:1)

Glossopharyngeal Neuralgia
    Male > Female

Head and Neck Cancer (US 1975–1998)

Type	Rate per 100,000 person-years	
	Male	Female
Lip	0.25	0.04
Tongue	1.51	0.99
Gum	1.06	1.00
Floor of Mouth	1.64	1.00
Other part of Mouth	1.27	0.91
Total Palate	2.09	1.41
Oropharynx	2.10	1.11
Tonsil	2.18	1.60
Nasopharynx	1.76	1.44
Pyriform Sinus	2.33	1.67
Hypopharynx	2.06	1.53
Other nonspecified oral/pharynx	2.31	1.35

Hearing Loss in Adult
    Male > Female (4:1)

Men incur more hearing loss than women from comparable noise exposure.

Juvenile Nasopharyngeal Angiofibroma
    Exclusively in boys

Keratoacanthoma of the External Ear
    Male > Female

Labyrinthitis
    Female > Male (1.5:1)

Laryngeal Carcinoma
    Male > Female (4–5:1)
    Except for postcricoid carcinomas, which are more frequent in women.
    A decrease in the male to female ratio noted since 1960 with an increase in the incidence of supraglottis lesions in women.
    Religious groups that forbid drinking and smoking have a low incidence of laryngeal cancer.
    Laryngoceles are found in 2% of healthy adults but 18% in patients with laryngeal cancer.

Leiomyosarcoma of the Larynx
    Male > Female
    Primarily in elderly men.

Lingual Thyroid
    Female > Male

Lip Cancer
    Male > Female (10–20:1)
    It is felt that lipstick may offer protection to females.
    88–98% occurs on the lower lip.

Liposarcoma of the Larynx
    Exclusively in men

Malignant Melanoma of the Face
    Male > Female (1.5:1)

Mastoiditis
    Male > Female

Melanoma of the Sinuses
    Male > Female

Motion Sickness
    Female > Male

Mouth Cancer
    Male > Female (1.5:1)

Nasal Polyps
    Male > Female (2:1)
    If asthma is present, the ratio is 1:1.

Nasal Septal Deviation
    Male > Female (2.7:1)

Nasopharyngeal Fibroma
    Male > Female

Nasopharyngeal Teratoma
    Female > Male (6:1)

Neurilemmoma of the Larynx
    Female > Male (slightly)

Oat Cell Carcinoma of the Larynx
    Male > Female (3:1)
    Associated with paraneoplastic syndromes.

Ossifying Fibroma
    Female > Male
    Primarily affects mandible.

Osteoma of Sinuses
    Male > Female
    80% occur in the frontal sinus.

Otitis Media
    Male > Female
    For acute and recurrent acute otitis media.
    Males are also more prone to middle ear effusion.

Otosclerosis
    Female > Male (2:1)
    It is clinically more common in females, although there is no difference in the incidence of histologic otosclerosis between sexes.

The onset usually occurs between 20–25 years of age, and rapid progression of hearing loss during or shortly after pregnancy occurs in about 50% of women.

Pharynx Cancer
    Male > Female (2.6:1)

Plummer-Vinson Syndrome
    Female > Male (9:1)
    Up to 30% of women with this condition develop postcricoid cancer.

Psychogenic Dysphonia
    Female > Male

Pterygopalatine Neuralgia
    Female > Male

Pyriform Sinus Carcinoma
    Male > Female (5:1)

Reinke's Edema
    Female > Male
    Usually in elderly smokers.

Rhabdomyosarcoma of the Larynx
    Male > Female (2:1)

Rhinophyma
    Male > Female

Salivary Gland Calculi
    Male > Female (2:1)

Salivary Gland Tumor
    Female > Male
        Pleomorphic Adenoma
    Female = Male
        Other adenomas

Sinonasal Tract Neoplasm
    Male > Female (2:1)
    Most are squamous cell carcinomas.

Sinusitis, Acute
    Female > Male (2:1)

Solitary Thyroid Nodule
    Female > Male (4:1)
    Solitary nodule in a male is likely cancerous.

Spasmodic Dysphonias
    Female > Male (3:2)

Stuttering
    Male > Female (3:1)
    Stuttering may represent a less stable neuromuscular control system for speech in boys, at least during the early years of development.

Subglottic Hemangioma
    Female > Male (2:1)

Temporomandibular Joint Syndrome
    Female > Male (3:1)

Thyroid Papillary Adenocarcinoma
    Female > Male (3:1)

Tongue Cancer
    Male > Female (1.9:1)

Tonsillar Squamous Cell Carcinoma
    Male > Female (2.5–3.5:1)
    Incidence is increasing in females.

Tracheomalacia/Laryngomalacia
    Male > Female (2:1)

Vasomotor Rhinitis
    Female > Male
        Especially elderly

Vestibular Schwannoma
    Female > Male (1.2:1)

Virilization of Voice
    Female > Male
    Often occurs after beginning hormone therapy.

Warthin's Tumor
    Male > Female
    Bilateral in 10% of the cases.

Winkler's Disease
    Male > Female (9:1)

X-Linked Hereditary Deafness Syndromes
    Male > Female
        Alport Syndrome
        Hunter Syndrome
        Oto-Palato Digital Syndrome
        Mixed Deafness and Perilymphatic Syndrome
        Gusher Syndrome
        Norrie Syndrome

Dental Health

Anatomy and Physiology

Mean Age (Years) at Eruption of Permanent Teeth

	Boys	Girls
Upper Jaw		
1st Incisor	7.22	6.94
2nd Incisor	8.42	8.01
Canine	10.09	10.42
1st Premolar	10.14	9.73
2nd Premolar	10.96	10.57
1st Molar	5.97	5.87
2nd Molar	11.81	11.37
Lower Jaw		
1st Incisor	6.26	6.08
2nd Incisor	7.35	6.99
Canine	10.42	9.58
1st Premolar	10.44	9.79
2nd Premolar	11.32	10.76
1st Molar	5.82	5.60
2nd Molar	11.45	10.93

Estimation of Calendar Age (Years) by Eruption of Teeth

Permanent Teeth	Boys	Girls	Error of Estimate
1 or 2 teeth	5.75	5.67	0.55
3 or 4 teeth	6.23	5.99	0.70
5 or 6 teeth	6.80	6.52	0.75
7 or 8 teeth	7.43	7.05	0.85
9 or 10 teeth	8.03	7.56	0.90
11 or 12 teeth	9.16	8.66	1.00

13 or 14 teeth	9.88	9.59	1.00
15 or 16 teeth	10.67	9.74	1.05
17 or 18 teeth	10.69	10.16	1.05
19 or 20 teeth	11.02	10.24	1.05
21 or 22 teeth	11.05	10.62	1.05
23 or 24 teeth	11.65	10.82	1.05
25 to 27 teeth	12.00	11.44	1.05

The vertical dimension of the mandibular rest position is greater in males than females. The growth velocity for the corpus length of the mandible is greater in boys than girls. The emergence of the deciduous dentition in boys is more precocious than in girls by about one month. This difference is present at the emergence of the upper central incisor and is maintained afterwards. The secretion rate of saliva is lower in females than in males.

Diseases

Alveolar Ridge Squamous Carcinoma
Female > Male

Apthous Stomatitis
Female > Male

Assymetric Mandibular Development
Male > Female
70% are male.

Behcet's Syndrome
Male > Female (2:1)

Burkitt's Lymphoma
Male > Female

Burning Mouth Syndrome
Female > Male (7–10:1)

Cherubism
Male > Female

Cleft Lip and Palate
Male > Female

Cleft Palate
    Female > Male

Coronoid Hyperplasia
    Male > Female

Discoid Lupus Erythematosus
    Female > Male

Eosinophilic Granuloma
    Male > Female (2:1)

Erythema Multiforme
    Female > Male (3:2)

Esophageal Tumor
    Male > Female

Geographic Tongue
    Female > Male (2:1)

Giant Cell Arteritis
    Female > Male

Hand-Schuller-Christian Disease
    Male > Female (2:1)

Hemangioma, Face/Oral
    Female > Male

Hiccups
    Male > Female (4:1)

Hodgkin's Disease
    Male > Female

Hypothyroidism
    Female > Male

Idiopathic Orofacial Pain
    Females > Males

Infectious Mononucleosis
    Peak age males: 18–23 years
    Peak age females: 15–16 years

Kaposi's Sarcoma
    Male > Female

Mal de Debarquement Syndrome
    Female > Male
    Usually occurs in middle aged females after an ocean cruise.

Malocclusion
    The neutral pattern occurs primarily in females, whereas most males demonstrate hypodivergent pattern.
    Males show a greater tendency toward prognathism, while females tend toward orthognathism and retrognathism.

Masticatory Muscle Pain
    Female > Male

Median Rhomboid Glossitis
    Female > Male (3–4:1)

Mitral Regurgitation, Rheumatic
    Female > Male (3:1)

Mitral Stenosis
    Female > Male (3:1)

Mitral Valve Prolapse
    Female > Male

Multiple Myeloma
    Male > Female

Muscular Dystrophy, Duchenne
    Male > Female

Myasthenia Gravis
    Female > Male

Osteitis Sicca
    Female > Male (8:1)

Osteomalacia
    Female > Male

Polyarteritis Nodosa
    Male > Female (2.5:1)

Prognathic Jaw
   Male > Female

Pyogenic Granuloma
   Female > Male (7:3)

Raynaud's Phenomenon
   Female > Male

Reiter's Syndrome
   Male > Female

Rheumatoid Arthritis
   Female > Male

Sjogren's Syndrome
   Female > Male

Speech Disorder
   Male > Female

Superficial Mucocoele
   Female > Male

Supernumery Deciduous Teeth
   Hyperdontia
      Male > Female (2:1)
   Mesiodens
      Male > Female (2:1)

Systemic Lupus Erythematosus
   Female > Male

Temporomandibular Joint Syndrome
   Female > Male (4:1)
   Primarily occurs in white females.
   Women that develop chronic TMJ syndrome are more likely to have a history of anxiety disorder compared to women that do not develop chronicity. This is not seen in men. However both males and females with chronic TMJ disorder have a greater frequency of depression.

Torus, Palate
   Female > Male (2:1)

Tracheitis
> Male > Female
> Primarily occurs in children.

Trigeminal Neuralgia
> Female > Male

Psychiatry

Anatomy and Physiology

The amygdala appears to handle emotionally charged memories in the right brain side of men and the left brain side of women. Men rely on the left inferior gyrus to carry out language tasks, whereas women use both the left and right inferior gyri to carry out the same task. Men and women carry out the task equally accurately and rapidly.

Body image: Males tend to see their bodies as functional and active and that need to be in shape and ready for use; while females view their body more in aesthetic and evaluative dimensions.

In early adolescence, increasing testosterone levels in boys has been associated with aggression, and changes in estrogen levels in girls has been associated with mood changes.

Pain: males tolerate acute pain better but females tolerate chronic pain better. Females are more sensitive than males to nociceptive stimuli including those that occur in internal organs. Kappa-opiod drugs are more effective analgesics in females than males.

Diseases

Addiction
    Females in treatment have lower self esteem and report more symptoms.
    Females have higher incidence of anxiety and depression with addiction than males.
    In females, addiction is associated with character pathology, eating disorders, post traumatic stress disorder and sexual abuse.

Alcoholism
- Males > Females (5:1)
- Lifetime risk for males 8–10%, for females 3–5%.
- Females are only half as likely to obtain treatment as compared to men.
- Females drink heavier later in life than males.
- Alcohol abuse and dependence progresses more rapidly in females.
- Females metabolize alcohol more slowly than men.
- Females develop higher blood alcohol concentration at a given dose of alcohol per kg of body weight compared to males.
- Females are more susceptible to medical complications related to drinking.
- Males are three times as likely to have alcohol-related problems recognized by their primary care doctor than are female drinkers.
- Some studies suggest alcoholism may have a greater genetic tendency in males.
- Women are more likely to die from all causes and alcohol-related liver disease than are men who report drinking the same amount of alcohol.
- Women develop alcoholic cirrhosis and hepatitis after a shorter period of heavy drinking and at a lower level of daily drinking than men.
- Female alcoholics have death rates 50–100% higher than male alcoholics (including deaths from suicides, alcohol-related accidents, circulatory disorders, and liver cirrhosis).
- Women become intoxicated after drinking smaller amounts of alcohol.
- Women have increased susceptibility to alcoholic liver disease, including fatty liver, hepatitis, and cirrhosis.
- Females who drink heavily may have increased susceptibility to neuropsychological impairment in a shorter length of time.
- Women appear to develop hypertension after short periods of heavy drinking.
- Women that drink heavily have a high mortality rate for most major alcohol related causes of death.

Alzheimers Dementia
- Female > Male

Amphetamine Abuse and Dependence
  Male > Female (3–4:1)
    IV use
  Male ≅ Female
    Non IV Use

Anorexia Nervosa
  Female > Male (9:1)
  About 1% of females in US have this condition.
  There is co-morbid major depression or dysthymia in 50–75% of cases.
  There is obsessive-compulsive disorder in 10–13% of cases.

Antisocial Personality Disorder
  Male > Female (3:1)

Anxiety
  Female > Male (2:1)
  Anxiety disorders often worsen premenstrually.
  Prevalence of anxiety conditions:
    Panic disorder: Female 3.2% Male 1.3%
    Agorophobia: Female > Male (8.5:1.5)
    Generalized Anxiety Disorder: Female > Male (3:2)
    Obsessive-Compulsive Disorder:
      Female 2.6–3.1%, Male 1.1–2.6%.
      Males tend to present at an earlier age. Modal age of onset for males is 6–15 years, for females 20–29 years.
    Agoraphobia with Panic Disorder: Female > Male (3:1)
    Simple Phobia: Female > Male (2:1)
    Specific Phobia: Varies with type
      Fear of heights: 55–70% Female
      Situational type: 75–90% Female
      Blood injection injury type: 55–70% Female
    Social Phobia: Female 5.2% Male 3.8%
      Female > Male in community studies.
      Male ≥ Female in clinical samples.
      Males are more likely to seek care for social phobia.
    Phobia to Animal or Nature:
      Females comprise 75–90% of cases
    Phobia to Blood: Females comprise 55–70% of cases
    Situational Fears: 75% are females

Anxiety Disorders
- Female > Male
    - 2–3x greater risk for Panic Disorder in females
    - Mitral valve prolapse often occurs together with panic attacks, especially in women.
- Female > Male
    - 2 x greater risk for Generalized Anxiety Disorder in females
- Female > Male
    - 2–3x greater risk for Specific Phobias in females
- Female > Male
    - Social Phobias
- Female = Male
    - In obsessive compulsive disorder; but obsessive compulsive disorder peaks out in childhood or adolescence for males but age 20's for females.

Asperger's Disorder
- Male > Female

Attention Deficit Hyperactivity Disorder
- Male > Female (3–9:1)
    - Children (some community studies find a 2:1 male to female ratio)
- Male = Female
    - Older adolescents
- Female > Male (2:1)
    - Young adults

Males with ADHD tend to have behavioral disturbances while females more likely to be disorganized and confused while remaining well behaved and quiet.

Atypical Depression
- Female > Male

Atypical Feature Specific Mood Disorder
- Female > Male (2–3:1)

Autism
- Male > Female (3–5:1)

Avoidant Personality Disorder
- Female = Male

Bereavement
Females present 3–4 times more than males for grief.

Binge Eating Disorder
Female > Male (1.5–2:1)

Bipolar Disorder
Female = Male
But, first episode in males is more likely a manic episode.
The first episode in females is usually major depressive episode.

Bipolar II Disorder
Female > Male

Body Dysmorphic Disorder
Female > Male (slightly)
Prevalence is increasing in men.
Muscle dysmorphia, a preoccupation that one's body is too small, is almost exclusive to men.

Borderline Personality Disorder
Female > Male (3:1)

Bulimia Nervosa
Female > Male (9:1)
Occurs in about 2–4% of females.

Caffeine Use
Male > Female

Cannabis Use Disorder
Male > Female

Child Abuse, Physical
Male > Female (3:2)

Child Abuse, Sexual
Female > Male (3:1)

Childhood Disintegrative Disorder
Male > Female

Cocaine Use Disorder
Male = Female

Conduct Disorder (Childhood Onset Type)
    Male > Female (2–3:1)

Conversion Disorder
    Female > Male (2–10:1)
    In females, symptoms are more common on the left side of the body. Females presenting with conversion disorder may later manifest full picture of somatization disorder.
    In males, an association with antisocial personality is evident.
    In men, conversion is often seen in the context of an industrial accident or military event.

Cyclothymic Disorder
    Female = Male
    But females are more likely to present for treatment.

Delirium Tremens
    Male > Female

Delusional Disorder
    Male = Female
        Overall
    Male > Female
        Jealous Type

Dependent Personality Disorder
    Female > Male

Depression, Major
    Female > Male
    Incidence 10% men, 20% women
    Prevalence 2.5% men, 8% women
    Males with depression have a 2–3 time increased chance of death compared to males without depression but no difference seen in women. Men tend to have more comorbid alcohol or drug abuse/dependence that tends to be chronic.
    Depressed men are apt to eat and sleep less and to feel agitated and to complete suicide; depressed women to eat and sleep more and feel persistent fatigue.
    Depressed women are more likely to report a greater number of symptoms, experience somatic anxiety symptoms and expressed

anger and to report increased appetite and weight gain and attempt suicide more than depressed men.

Men tend to worry about the impact on job performance and finances, and attempt to cope by distracting themselves from their feelings.

Women tend to worry about the impact on family and other close relationships, and more likely to brood instead of denying their feelings.

Among those with unipolar and bipolar disorders, women are more likely to have periods of rapid cycling from depression to mania or hypomania.

Women manifest more seasonality in their timing of depression. Depression is more likely to occur in the winter in women.

Women also have periods of increased risk for mood disorders such as during the postpartum period.

Females also seem more vulnerable for the onset of major depression during the luteal phase of the cycle.

Prior anxiety is associated with increased risk for depression in both sexes but women with depression are more likely to report a history of anxiety disorders.

Some studies show that depressed females have increased cortisol secretion compared to control females but this difference was not found in depressed men.

When deprived of tryptophan, a precursor of serotonin, serotonin synthesis drops four times more in females. This may partially explain the higher rates of depression in women.

Men with depression are more likely to have stress intolerance, low impulse control, alcohol misuse, and aggressive behavior.

During stressful times, most women with breast cancer want to talk about it and share their feelings with others, but most men with prostate cancer would rather not.

Men in support groups prefer to share information, whereas women prefer to share emotions.

Dissociative Disorder
    Female > Male (2–9:1)
        Adults
    Female = Male
        Children
    Females average 15 identities, males average 8.

Domestic Violence
> Females suffer more episodes than males.
> Increased risk for alcohol abuse in females suffering domestic violence and psychiatric illness rate higher in women.

Down's Syndrome
> Male > Female (1.3:1)

Drug Abuse
> Women are more prone to become addicted to prescription antidepressants and sedatives and to combine them with alcohol as a coping mechanism.
>
> Women appear to become more dependent after using marijuana, heroin and cocaine for a shorter period of time than men.
>
> Women seem less sensitive to cocaine than men. Men experience more euphoria and dysphoria and detect cocaine's effects sooner than women. Women in treatment for cocaine use are more likely to report negative emotions and interpersonal problems before they relapse.
>
> Women are more likely to be impulsive in their return to using cocaine. Men are more likely to report positive emotions prior to relapse.
>
> Men in drug treatment programs are more likely to relapse than women, partly because women engage in group counseling more often.
>
> Women that smoke tobacco tend to smoke fewer cigarettes a day, inhale less deeply and smoke lower nicotine-containing cigarettes. However females have more trouble quitting smoking, may experience more severe withdrawal, and appear to gain more weight after quitting than men.
>
> Daughters, but not sons, of women that smoked during pregnancy are more likely to smoke.

Dysthymic Disorder
> Female > Male (2–3:1)
>> In adults
>
> Female = Male
>> Children

Eating Disorder
> Female > Male

75% of females perceive fatness although the percentage of being overweight is actually similar between the sexes. This reflects differences in the social learning process of how to view personal weight.

Females tend to be dissatisfied with their body from the waist down, while in males it is from the waist up.

Females tend to be more concerned with weight than shape but the opposite is true in men.

75–80% of females desire weight loss, but in males 40% desire weight loss and 40% desire weight gain.

Males tend to have more specific goals behind weight loss than females.

Males are more likely to suffer from reverse anorexia or fear of being thin and a drive to bulk up.

Female > Male (up to 10:1)
    Anorexia Nervosa
        White > Nonwhite

Female > Male (10–20 times)
    Bulimia Nervosa
        White > Nonwhite

Encopresis
    Male > Female (1.5:1)
        In children, boys are 3–6 times more likely to have condition.

Enuresis
    Male > Female

Expressive Language Disorder, Developmental
    Male > Female

Factitious Disorder
    Male > Female

Factitious Disorder by Proxy
    Female > Male
        As perpetrator

Fetal Alcohol Syndrome
    Especially high in Eskimos.
    Females have higher blood alcohol levels and become more intoxicated when given the same amount of alcohol.

There is decreased activity of alcohol dehydrogenase in the female stomach.

Fragile-X Syndrome
80% of males and 65% of females have IQ's less than 70.
Males more severely affected.
Females have higher carrier rate.

Gender Identity Disorder
Male > Female (3–5:1)

Hallucinogen Use
Male > Female (3:1)

Histrionic Personality Disorder
Female > Male

Hypochondriasis
Male = Female
But females are more likely to seek medical attention.

Inhalant Abuse
Male > Female
70–80% are male.

Insomnia
Female > Male

Intermittent Explosive Disorder
Male > Female

Klein-Levin Syndrome of Primary Hypersomnia
Male > Female (3:1)

Kleptomania
Female > Male

Korsakoff's Psychosis
Males > Females
Most common in alcoholics.

Major Depressive Disorder
Female > Male (2:1)

Major Depressive Episode
Female > Male (2:1)

Mental Retardation
Male > Female (1.5:1)

Mixed Episode Mood Disorder
Male > Female

Mixed Receptive-Expresssive Language Disorder (Developmental)
Male > Female

Mood Disorders
Depression, mood disturbances, mood cycling, and loss reactions are more prevalent in women.
Increased mood or somatic changes are noted premenstrually.

Munchausen's Syndrome
Male > Female (2:1)

Narcissitic Personality Disorder
Male > Female (2–3:1)

Neuroleptic Induced Tardive Dyskinesis
Female > Male
   Elderly
Female = Male
   Young

Neuroleptic Malignant Syndrome
Male > Female

Nicotine Use
Male > Female
Rapidly increasing in females.

Nightmare Disorder
Male > Female (2–4:1)

Obsessive-Compulsive Personality Disorder
Male > Female (1–2:1)
Early onset is more common in males. (Age 17 years in males and age 21 years in females)
Later onset form is more common in females.

Opioid Abuse
Male > Female (3–4:1)

Oppositional Defiant Disorder
- Male > Female
  - Before puberty
- Male = Female
  - After puberty

Pain Disorder
- Female > Male
- Especially for headache and musculoskeletal pain in females. Females have a larger variety of coping strategies than males.

Panic Disorder
- Female > Male (3:1)

Paranoid Personality Disorder
- Male > Female

Paraphilia
- Male > Female

Pathologic Gambling Disorder
- Male > Female (2:1)

PCP Abuse
- Male > Female (2:1)

Pedophilia
- Male > Female (4–9:1)
- In males, about 75% attracted to females exclusively, 25% attracted to males exclusively, and a small percent attracted to both sexes.

Perinatal Loss
- Females grieve more than males.
- Prolonged depression may occur in 25% of females.

Phobias
- Female > Male
  - Overall

Phobia, Social
- Female > Male
- Community studies, but Male $\geq$ Female in clinical studies

Phonological Disorder
- Male > Female

Postconcussional Disorder
   Male > Female

Post-Psychotic Depressive Disorder of Schizophrenia
   Female = Male

Post-Traumatic Stress Disorder
   Females > Male (2:1)
   Adult women more likely to ask for help.
   Most men with PTSD have experienced combat or trauma on the job. Most women have a history of rape or physical assault.
   PTSD tends to last longer in females.
   Probabilty of PTSD in women versus men exposed to assault was 36% in women and 6% in men.
   Lifetime prevalence of PTSD is about 5–6% of males and 10–14% of females.
   Traumatic event exposure is higher in males as is the proportion with history of multiple exposures to traumatic events.
   The risk of PTSD associated with traumatic event exposure is 6.2% in males and 13% in females.
   Females have higher risk of PTSD in connection with being held captive, tortured, kidnapped, sexually assaulted (other than rape), mugged, held up, badly beaten or threatened with a weapon.

Primary Insomnia
   Male > Female

Psychiatric Disorders
   In general, women experience more comorbid illnesses, have a higher rate of disability and morbidity, and suffer more often from reversible drug-induced or medically induced psychiatric conditions.

Pyromania
   Male > Female

Rape Crisis Syndrome
   Female > Male

Rapid Cycling Specific Mood Disorder
   Female > Male
   70–90% are female.

Reading Disorders
    Male > Female (2:1)
    60–80% are male.

Receptive Language Disorder
    Male > Female

Retts Disorder
    Females only

Rumination Disorder
    Male > Female

Schizoaffective Disorder
    Female > Male

Schizoid Personality Disorder
    Male > Female

Schizophrenia
    Male > Female (1–2:1)
    Onset is earlier in males (15–24 years) than females (25–34 years). More severely affects cognitive function in males and isn't as amenable to treatment in males.
    The inferior parietal lobe in male schizophrenics is smaller on the left than the right (normally larger on the left) and 16% smaller than normal (No significant differences seen in female schizophrenics).
    Females experience a later onset, less disability, and an increased benefit from drug therapy.
    The prolactin response to neuroleptic drugs is greater in females.
    Schizophrenic females more likely to express dysphoria, persecutory delusions and a higher family morbidity risk for schizophrenia than schizophrenic men.

Schizotypal Personality Disorder
    Male > Female

Seasonal Affective Disorder
    Female > Male (4:1)

Seasonal Pattern Specific Mood Disorder
    Female > Male
    60–90% are female.

Sedative, Prescription Hypnotic or Anxiolytic Disorder
Female > Male

Selective Mutism
Female > Male

Separation Anxiety Disorder
Female > Male

Sexual Abuse
Childhood
Female: 27–38%
Males: 7–10%

Shared Psychotic Disorder
Female > Male

Sleep Disorder Related to Another Mental Disorder
Female > Male
Sleep studies show females have higher total sleep requirements than males.

Sleep Problems
Female > Male
Women are twice as likely to report difficulty initiating sleep, more awakenings, and poor sleep quality.

Sleep Terror Disorder
Male > Female
Childhood
Male = Female
Adult

Somatization Disorder
Female > Male (up to 10:1)
Occurs in 0.25%–2.0% in women, < 0.2% in men.
More common in women in the United States; more common in males in other countries.

Stereotypic Movement Disorder
Male > Female (3:1)
Headbanging
Female > Male
Self-biting

Stuttering
> Male > Female (3:1)

Substance Abuse Disorder
> Male > Female
> Overall, but varies with the class of substance.
> Females usually begin using substances later than do men, are strongly influenced by spouses or boyfriends to use, and enter treatment earlier in their course of substance use.
> Women also have more comorbid psychiatric disorders such as depression and anxiety and they are usually preexisting.
>> Alcohol
>>> Male > Female
>>> Lifetime prevalence of 17.9% in females, 35.4% in males. Females drink less alcohol, begin at a later age and develop pattern of abuse at a later age. Women are more likely to date onset to stressful event, drink more often solitary, and are more likely to be divorced when they enter addiction treatment.
>>> In seeking treatment, women are more likely to be motivated by health and family problems, vs. job and legal problems for men.
>> Smoking
>>> Males > Female
>>> Women are less successful in quitting than men.
>>> Blacks are less successful in quitting than whites.
>> Other
>>> Women abuse prescription drugs more than men.
>>> Women use illicit drugs less than men.
>>> Women suffer greater societal stigma for their addiction.

Substance-Induced Sexual Dysfunction
> Male > Female
> Orgasmic disorder more common in men.

Suicide
> Male > Female (3–4:1)
>> Completed
> Female > Male (3:1)
>> Attempted

Tourette's Disorder
    Male > Female (1.5–3:1)

Tourette's Syndrome
    Male > Female (3–9:1)

Trichotillomania
    Female > Male

Undifferentiated Somatiform Disorder
    Female > Male

Vascular Dementia
    Male > Female

Wernicke's Encephalopathy
    Male > Female

Behavioral and Psychological Health

Activity Patterns

Time spent on various activities of men and women in the US

Activity	Hours per week (rounded)	
	Male	Female
Time spent at home	103	119
Time away from home	52	38
Time Traveling	12	10
Job related	36	18
House/yard	9	20
Child Care	1	4
Services/Shopping	3	6
Personal Care	77	79
Education	2	1
Organizations	3	3
Social Activity	8	9
Leisure	29	28

Males and females differ in their hobbies. Among the top 10 hobbies, only bowling was shared between the sexes.

Behavioral Patterns of US Students and Adults

Behavior Characteristics of Alternative High School Students

Females less likely to attend an alternative high school than male students (44% vs. 55%). Of students at alternative high schools, females are more likely to wear a motorcycle helmet, more likely to wear seatbelts, but less likely to drive after drinking. Males are 3–4 times more likely to carry a weapon and also more likely to be in a physical fight and about twice as likely injured in a physical fight as females. Males attending alternative schools are more likely to currently use marijuana or cocaine. However white females were as likely to be lifetime cocaine users as white males. Males were also slightly more likely to use steroids illegally and sniff or inhale toxic substances. Males were more likely to begin using illicit substances before age 13 years than females. Males are more likely to initiate sexual intercourse before age 13 years and have >3 partners during their lifetime. Males are also less likely to talk to their parents about AIDS or HIV. Males are more likely to eat >2 high fat foods daily. Females more likely to report suicide ideation, not use a condom during intercourse, eat < 5 fruits/vegetables daily, use laxatives or vomiting or take diet pills to lose weight or keep from gaining weight. Females are less likely to participate in vigorous physical activity.

*Behavior Characteristics of US College Students
18–24 years old (1995)*

Seat belt use
> 14% of males and 8.4% of females never or rarely use seat belts when riding in a car. When driving a car 13.2% of males and 6.4% of females rarely or never use seatbelts.

Helmet use
> 34.1% of males and 41.1% of females rarely or never wear helmet riding a motorcycle and 88.7% of males and 89.8% of females never or rarely use a helmet when riding a bicycle.

Drinking and Recreation
> 41.4% of males and 36.6% of females had ridden with a driver that had been drinking.
> 32.7% of males and 23.2% of females had drunk alcohol and driven a vehicle before.

33.2% of males and 23.7% of females had been drinking while boating or swimming.

Carried a Weapon during the Last Month
14.1% of males and 3.4% of females

Ever had Sexual Intercourse
77.8% of males and 81% of females

Currently Sexually Active (during the last 3 months)
56.8% of males and 66.8% of females

> 5 Sex Partners during Lifetime
27.8% of males and 23.9% of females

Ever Been Forced to have Sexual Intercourse
3.6% of males and 17% of females

Contraceptive Use during Last Sexual Intercourse
Male: 82.3%, Female: 88.8%

Alcohol or Drug Use during Last Sexual Intercourse
26.6% of males and 14% of females

Been Pregnant or got Someone Pregnant
11.4% of females and 15.1% for males

Been in a Physical Fight during the Last 12 Months and Needed Treatment for Injury
9% of females had been in a physical fight and 0.5% of them were treated.
17.7% of males had been in a fight and 1.2% treated for injury.

Current Tobacco or Smokeless-Tobacco Use
36.7% of males smoked tobacco and 13.6% used smokeless variety.
29.1% of females smoked and 0.5% used smokeless-tobacco.

Current Alcohol Use
73.2% of males had drunk at least once during the last month and 5.4% drunk on at least 20 days during the last month.
67% of females had drunk at least once during the last month and 1.6% drank for at least 20 days of the last month.

Current Marijuana Use
20.3% of males and 14.7% of females had used at least once during the last month.

Current Cocaine Use
  1.3% of males and 0.6% of females had used cocaine within the last month.

Current Illegal Drug Use
  4.6% of males and 2.2% of females currently use illegal drugs.
  Lifetime illegal drug use was 17.6% of males and 14.7% for females.

Lifetime Inhalant Use
  11.7% of males and 7.7% of females

Lifetime Illegal Steroid Use
  2% of males and 0.3% of females

Lifetime Injecting Drug Use
  1.3% of males and 0.2% of females

Ate > 4 Servings of Fruits and Vegetables on the Day Before the Survey
  23.2% of females and 27% of males

Ate < 3 Servings of Foods Typically High in Fats on the Day Before the Survey
  84.6% of females and 65.9% of males

Thought they were Overweight
  41.8% of females and 26.5% of males

Attempting Weight Loss by Various Means
  Attempting weight loss
    26.2% of males and 59% of females
  Dieting
    14% of males and 40.5% of females
  Exercising
    41.7% of males and 64.3% of females
  Vomiting or laxatives
    5.1% of females and 0.4% of males
  Took diet pills
    6.4% of females and 0.8% of males

Engaged in Physical Activity
  Vigorous
    48.9% of males and 35.3% of females

Moderate
: 19.6% of males and 20.8% of females

Stretching exercises
: 36% for both sexes

Strengthening exercises
: 37.1% of males and 30% of females

Behavioral Characteristics of US Civilian, Noninstitutionalized Adults (age > 18) in 1996 and 1997

Report being Overweight
- Men: approximately 61%
- Women: approximately 44.3%

Report No Leisure Time Activity
- Women: 30.8%
- Men: 26%

Current Cigarette Use
- Women: 21.4%
- Men: 25.4%

Binge Drinking
- Men: 22.3%
- Women: 6.7%

Chronic Drinking
- Men: 5.4%
- Women: 0.8%

Drinking and Driving
- Men: 3%
- Women: 0.9%

Seat-Belt Use (always wear)
- Men: 62%
- Women: 75%

Hypertension Awareness
- Men: 22.3%
- Women: 23.6%

Diabetes Awareness
    Men: 4.2%
    Women: 4.7%

High Cholesterol Awareness
    Men: 27.9%
    Women: 28.8%

Ever Had Cholesterol Checked
    Men: 70.8%
    Women: 76.7%

Ever had Sigmoidoscopy or Proctoscopy (age >50 years)
    Men: 45.3%
    Women: 37.7%

Ever had Fecal Occult Blood Test (age > 50 years)
    Men: 16.8%
    Women: 19.5%

Ever had Pneumococcal Vaccine (age > 65 years)
    Men: 44.3%
    Women: 46.9%

Influenza Vaccine in the Previous Year (age > 65 years)
    Men: 67.9%
    Women: 65.5%

Having No Health Insurance
    Men: 15.2%
    Women: 13.5%

Cost as a Barrier to Health Care
    Men: 9.1%
    Women: 13.4%

Other Psychological and Behavioral Differences

Bereavement
    Females present to psychiatrists 3–4 times more often than males for grief.

With perinatal loss, females grieve more than males and prolonged depression may occur in 25% of females.

Cognitive Abilities

Women demonstrate an advantage in verbal abilities, particularly verbal fluency, speech production, the ability to decode a language and spelling, perceptual speed and accuracy and fine motor skills. Men show an advantage on tests of spatial abilities, quantitative abilities, target directed motor skills, and gross motor strength.

Females have an advantage in remembering both verbal and non-verbal information.

Men outperform women in the manipulation of spatial information and navigating a route.

Men perform better in test of target-directed motor skills, i.e. in guiding or intercepting projectiles.

Females remember visual information better.

Females perform better on test that measure word recall and on test to find words that begin with a certain letter or fulfill some other constraint. They are better than men at rapidly identifying matching items and in landmark memory.

Female sex hormones appear to enhance performance skills that are usually done better by females whereas they cause a decrement in performance of those skills usually done better by males.

Women's performances at certain tasks change throughout the menstrual cycle.

When using some abstract verbal skills, women do use both hemispheres of the brain more equally than men.

Males are better at technical drawing.

Males and females navigate routes differently.

Competition

Blood levels of testosterone rise when a male is about to compete. The winner's testosterone level continues to rise after the event while the loser's falls.

Males are more aggressive than females, whereas young females are more nurturing and engage in less rough and tumble activities than young boys.

Diet

Women consume a lower percentage of beef (14%) and pork (7%) than men (18% and 9% respectively).

Women consume a higher percentage of poultry (13%), dairy (22%) and fruit and vegetables (11%) than men (11%, 19% and 9% respectively).

Obesity, defined as a body mass index ≥ 30 kg/m^2 was present in 18.1% of females and 17.7% of males in 1998. The prevalence has increased about 6% in both sexes since 1991.

Men tend to exercise more than women.

Men tend to carry their weight at the waistline (apple shape) and women on their hips and thighs (pear shape).

Abdominal obesity in men is riskier than lower-body obesity in women.

Domestic Violence

Females suffer more episodes than males.

Increased risk of alcohol abuse in females suffering domestic violence and psychiatric illness rates are higher in females.

Emotion Recognition

Males are more likely to have difficulty recognizing one emotion from another based on facial expression.

Group Interactions

Males are more hierarchal than females, while females are more egalitarian.

Males are easier to train because of group cooperation.

Females deal better with people.

Health Care Concerns

While women constitute 52% of the US population they make 57% of the visits to doctors, are prescribed 60% of all prescriptions, and undergo 59% of hospital procedures.

Women make 75% of health care decisions and spend 2 of every 3 health care dollars.

Women use more conventional medicine and alternative medicine services than men. Women also use more homeopathic remedies.

Women spend 35% more time confined to bed.

Health Knowledge

Females are more knowledgeable about health.

Females are more aware of their blood pressure, cholesterol and diabetes status than males.

Females are slightly more likely to have had pneumomococcal vaccination than men. (37.7% vs. 35.3%).

Women are more diligent about checkups and preventive care.

A recent survey found that 76% of women had been tested for health problems in the last year compared to 64% of men.

Language

Male language asserts superiority. It emphasizes and promotes the self whereas women more frequently use language to draw out others and to include them.

Male language seeks to establish power and dominance over other people while women's language minimizes status differences and promotes equality.

Quality of Life

Of patients with arthritis, females report 8.9 days within the last 30 days as being unhealthy compared to 7.8 days for men with arthritis.

For patients without arthritis, females report 4.5 vs. 3.2 unhealthy days for males during the preceding 30 days.

Risk Takers

Males are less likely to wear seatbelts by 15%.

Males are more likely to drive drunk (3.7% males and 0.9% female).

Males are less likely to wear sunscreen.

90% of on the job fatalities are men.

5 out of 7 victims of traffic accidents are male.

4 of 5 homicides are male.

4 of 5 suicides are male.

Most responsibility on contraception is placed on women but half of sexually active girls between 13–44 years of age do not always use birth control.

Males are more likely to binge drink (21.3% vs. 6.9%).

Males are more likely to work outdoors but females are more likely to sunbathe.

Young men tend to seek immediate rewards more so over larger but later ones.

Young men are more likely to escalate an altercation to a higher, potentially lethal level.

Self-Esteem
> Adolescence seems to be more difficult for females. They report more depression, dissatisfaction with their bodies, eating disorders, and lower self-esteem by the time they reach high school compared to males. Female adolescents also have more negative assessments of their intellectual abilities than males.
>
> These findings may explain why girls have higher incidence of suicide attempts, depression, and eating disorders.
>
> Maturation in boys is associated with added status and positive self-esteem but with lower self-esteem, and lower scholastic self-perception in girls.

Stress
> Females more likely to report stress in comparable life stages and under similar circumstances than men.
>
> Female catecholamine and blood pressure tend to stay elevated for a longer period of time after leaving a stressful workday.
>
> Females are slightly less likely to report leisure time activity.
>
> Type A behavior tends to be more common in males.
>
> Women tend to be more aware of their own feelings and the feelings of others than men are.
>
> Men are more sensitive to the depressogenic effects of divorce or separation and work problems.
>
> Women are more sensitive to the depressogenic effects of problems getting along with people in their proximal network.
>
> Women report more interpersonal whereas men report more legal and work related stressful life events.

Sexual Abuse, Childhood
> Female > Male
>> Males 7–10%
>> Females 27–38%

Pharmacology/Toxicology

Anatomy and Physiology

Anatomic and Physiologic Parameters for Males and Nonpregnant Females

Parameter	Adult Male	Adult Female
Body Surface Area	18,000 cm^2	16000 cm^2
Total Body Water	42 L	29 L
Extracellular Water	18.2 L	11.6 L
Intracellular Water	23.8 L	17.4 L
Minute Volume Ventilation	7.5 L/min	6.0 L/min
Respiratory Rate	15 breaths/min	15 breaths/min
Volume of Air Exchanged in 8 Hours	3600 L	2900 L
Total Lung Capacity	5.6 L	5.0 L
Functional Residual Capacity	3.1 L	2.8 L
Ventilatory Capacity	4.3 L	3.3 L
Volume of Distribution	160 ml	130 ml
Total Volume (ml/breath)	750	487

Physiologic Parameters that Affect Absorption and Distribution and Metabolism

Parameter	Difference (Male (M) vs. Female (F))
Gastric Juice pH	M > F for acidity (pH 1.92 vs. 2.59)
Gastric Juice Flow	M > F
Intestinal Motility	M > F
Gastric Emptying	M > F
Dermal Thickness	M > F
Pulmonary Function	M > F
Cardiac Output	M > F

Gut Transit Time	44.8 hours in males vs. 91.7 hours in females
Plasma Volume	M > F
Total Body Water	M > F
Body Fat	F > M
Basal Metabolic Rate	Higher BMR in males increases metabolism
Renal Blood Flow	M > F

Cardiac Output (CO) to Organs Differs for Certain Body Sites

Tissue	% CO in Males	% CO In Females
Adipose	5%	8.5%
Heart	4%	5%
Kidney	19%	17%
Liver	25%	27%
Muscle	17%	12%

Median Total Body Surface Area (m^2) for Humans By Age

Age (Years)	Males	Females
3–5	0.728	0.711
6–8	0.931	0.919
9–11	1.16	1.16
12–14	1.49	1.48
15–17	1.75	1.60
Adult	1.94	1.69

Dietary and Pharmocologic Differences in Males and Females

Total fluid intake in men is 1.8–2.2 liters/day; in women 1.5–1.6 liters per day. Women eat more fruit but less fish and vegetables than men. Meat, dairy and grain consumption tends to be higher in males. Women eat less food than men and may have more difficulty getting enough nutrients. Women are more likely to have lower intakes of iron, zinc, magnesium, protein and calcium than men. Women are disproportionately affected by iodine deficiency and goiter as well. Women diet more often and consume more low fat foods and beverages. Women get about 32% of their calories from fat while men get about 44% of their daily calories from fat. The concentration of total ascorbic acid is higher in females than in males. Elderly females have a higher BMI and a lower waist-to-hip ratio than elderly males. Older females reduce their food intake compared to young females much less than do older men compared to young men. Older females are more likely to take vitamin or mineral supplements than older males. Extracellular and intracellular water volumes are smaller in females. Women have more adipose tissue (32% vs. 21%), less skeletal muscle, (29% vs. 40% of body weight), and lower skin weight (3.1% vs. 3.7%) than men. Females have a longer gastric emptying time and secrete less gastric acid, and the intestinal transit time is often slower in females. This affects absorption and bioavailabilty of some drugs. The total body water value is 40% higher in men, whereas the percentage body fat is higher in women. Thus the plasma concentration of lipophilic drugs may be lower in females at the same dosage. Renal function and clearance depend on body weight, body surface area, age and gender. Men have higher serum and urinary creatinine levels and higher creatinine clearance values. Thus the dosage of renally excreted drugs may be different between sexes. The epidermis on the arms and fingers is slightly thicker in males and may affect transcutaneous absorption. Because women have more body fat they may store more fat soluble toxic material even if exposed to the same dose as men. Female hormones have been proposed to increase susceptibility to toxins by deregulating growth and differentiation via receptor binding.

Women have a shallower ventilatory response to hypercapnia than males. Progesterone modulates the sensitivity to rising CO_2 with lowest resting arterial CO_2 seen during the luteal phase. Xanthine oxidase activity tends to be lower in males. Uridine Diphosphate Glucuronosyl transferase activity appears to be higher in males.

Side chain oxidation and glucuronidation are increased by testosterone in men (perhaps women) but ring oxidation is not. Men have higher levels of glucuronosyl transferase. Women appear to have higher incidence of polymorphisms in certain genes related to Phase II metabolism and in the p53 tumor suppressor gene. Sex hormones affect the potassium channels: estrogen has a down-regulating effect on K-channel activity.

The regulation of the sympathetic nervous system (SNS) in females is altered such that sympatho-adrenal activation is attenuated or inhibition is augmented. Pathways regulating the SNS appear to be less sensitive to excitatory stimuli in females. Females have greater baroreflex sensitivity such that alterations in blood pressure are more efficiently controlled than in males. Cardiopulmonary reflex inhibition of sympathetic nerve activity is greater in females. Females appear to have an attenuated sensitivity to adrenergic nerve stimulation, but not to noradrenaline. Females have an attenuated stress-induced increase in plasma catecholamines suggesting that females are less sensitive or less responsive to adrenal medullary activation.

Hepatic metabolism may be affected by gender as some isoenzymes are male specific or regulated by male hormones. Hepatic glucuronidation is often decreased in females, thus increasing the half-life of some drugs in women. The use of oral contraceptives by women may alter hepatic metabolism.

Women experience more cycles of fat loss and gain because of dieting and pregnancy. If toxicants stored in tissue are mobilized during these periods, this could be a significant factor. Overall women tend to have greater bioavailability and slower clearance of drugs compared to men, the consequence being that correct doses in males may be relatively high for females. The majority of studies have found that there is a 28–36% decrease in the rate of gastric emptying premenstrually. There may be a significant decline in renal clearance between the luteal and early follicular phase.

Pregnancy Effects on Drug Concentrations

Pregnancy affects the way drugs are handled in women. Drug absorption is altered as gastric emptying is reduced, and a 40% decrease in gastric acid secretion and 30–40% drop in pepsin activity occurs. Intestinal motility increases and pulmonary tidal volume increases. The volume of distribution for drugs changes as plasma volume increases by 50% while total body water increases by 7–8 liters and body fat increases 20–40% during pregnancy. Plasma drug concentrations may be altered due to decline in albumin levels, while free fatty acid and lipoprotein values increase in pregnancy. Metabolism and elimination are also altered due to higher levels of hormones affecting hepatic drug metabolism, whereas oxidative metabolism declines prolonging half-life of some drugs. Renal function and clearance rise increasing the elimination of many drugs and reducing concentrations in pregnant females.

Cytochrome Enzyme Differences between the Sexes

CYP3A4 activity is greater in younger women than in men and postmenopausal women. Females have 20–50% higher activity of CYP3A4. An age-related decrease in CYP3A4 metabolism occurs to a greater extent in males.

CYP1A and CYP2C19 activity is less in females.

CYP2D6 activity is similar by sex but CYP2D6 decreases during the luteal phase when estrogen levels are peaking. CYP2D6 activity may decline after ovariectomy.

Drugs metabolized by CYP3A4 are extensively cleared by females whereas drugs cleared by other isozymes are usually cleared faster by males.

CYP3A4activity is regulated by estrogen and progesterone at the gene level.

CYP1A2 activity is higher in males.

CYP2E1 activity is higher in males.

CYP2C19 activity is higher in males.

Vitamin Recommended Daily Allowances (RDAs) for Adults

Vitamin	RDA for Male	RDA for Female
Vitamin A	5000 IU	4000 IU
Thiamine	1.5 mg	1.1 mg
Riboflavin	1.7 mg	1.3 mg
Niacin	19 mg	15 mg
Pyridoxine	2 mg	1.6 mg
Folic acid	200 mcg	180 mcg
Cobalamin	2 mcg	2 mcg
Vitamin C	60 mg	60 mg
Vitamin D	5 mcg	5 mcg
Vitamin E	15 IU	12 IU
Vitamin K	80mcg	65 mcg

Pharmocodynomic/Pharmocokinetic Differences in Males and Females for Certain Drugs

Drug Class	Drug	Differences seen in Female (F) vs Male (M)
Analgesics	Aspirin	Longer half-life in F
	Nalbuphine	Greater analgesic efficacy in F
	Pentazocine	Greater analgesic efficacy in F
	Butorphanol	Greater analgesic efficacy in F
	Morphine	Greater analgesic efficacy in F
	Ibuprofen	Less analgesic efficacy in F
	Naproxen	Clearance slower in F
	Acetaminophen	Clearance slower in F
	Diclofenac	Higher activity in F
	Piroxicam	Greater clearance in M

Antiasthmatics	Theophylline	Shorter half-life by 33% in F
Antibiotics	Erythromycin	Increased rate of metabolism in F
		Increased QT interval in F
		Increased risk of Torsades de pointes in F
		Increased plasma clearance in F
		CO_2 breath tests 37% higher in F
	Rifampicin	Increased rate of absorption in F
	Cefataxime	Decreased clearance in F
	Amantadine	Renal excretion inhibited by quinidine and quinine in M, not F
Anticonvulsants	Phenytoin	Increased levels in F
	Mephabarbital	Decreased clearance in F
	Mephenytoin	Greater clearance in F
Antidepressants	Imipramine	Increased levels by 63% in F
	Clomipramine	Increased levels by 63% in F
	Trazadone	Increased volume of distribution in F
		Decreased clearance in elderly M
	Sertraline	Longer half-life and higher plasma levels in F
	Fluvoxamine	Increased levels by 40–50% in F
	Nortriptyline	Plasma conc 1.3 times higher in F
	Lithium	Thyroid toxicity 5 fold higher in F
	Nefazodone	Higher plasma levels in elderly F
Barbiturates	Phenobarbital	Increased levels in F
	Methylphe-nobarbital	Greater clearance in M
Benzodiazepines	Chlor-diazepoxide	Longer half-life, greater volume of distribution in F
	Oxazepam	Longer half-life (1.3 times) in F
	Diazepam	Longer half-life in young F
	Nitrazepam	Unbound concentrations higher in F
	Lorazepam	T1/2 Male > Female (1.3 fold)
	Midazolam	Clearance faster in F
	Desmethyl-diazepam	Clearance higher in M

Cardiovascular	Lidocaine	Longer half life in F
	Propanolol	Increased levels, decreased clearance in F
		C2C19 dependent side chain hydoxylation higher in M
	Amlodipine	Better hypotensive response in F
	Hydralazine	Increased incidence of lupus in F
	Coumadin	Increased levels in F
	Quinidine	Greater QT prolongation in F
	Sotalol	Increased risk of Torsades de Pointes in F
	Disopyramide	Increased risk of Torsades de Pointes in F
	Amiodarone	Increased risk of Torsades de Pointes in F
	Bepridil	Increased risk of Torsades de Pointes in F
	Prenylamine	Increased risk of Torsades de Pointes in F
	Ibutilide	Increased risk of Torsades de Pointes in F
	Mibefradil	Increased rhabdomyolysis in F
	K+ Channel Blockers	Increased risk of Torades de Pointes in F
	Isoproterenol	M show significant dose response to vasodilation, F do not
	Verapamil	Increased clearance in F
	Digoxin	Decreased clearance in F
	Labetolol	Higher plasma levels in F
Hypolipidemics	Cerivastatin	Maximum concentrations higher and increased risk of myopathy I in elderly F
	Probucol	Increased risk of Torsades de Pointes and tachyarrhythmias in F
OTHERS	Caffeine	Increase clearance in F
	Ethanol	Decreased first-pass metabolism in F
		Peak acetaldehyde higher in M

	after an acute dose of alcohol
	Sedative effects greater in F
Vitamin C	Increased clearance in F
Iron	Better absorption in preadolescent girls
Oral contraceptives	Induce glucuronidation in F
Propanolol	Decreased clearance in F
Vecuronium	Higher plasma concentrations in F
Mephenytoin	Increased activity/clearance in F
Methylphenobarbital	Decreased clearance in F
Piroxicam	Decreased clearance in F
Tacrine	Increased levels in F
Clozapine	Increased levels in F
Fluvoxamine	Increased levels in F
Aspirin	Appears to thin blood better in M
Antipyrine	Faster half-life in F
Cocaine	F have only 1/2 of the plasma level after the same initial dose
Quinine	F more likely to develop drug induced TTP-HUS syndrome
Imipramine	Unbound concentrations higher in F
ACE Inhibitors	F more likely to develop cough
Aloestron	Ineffective in males with IBS
Sertraline	More effective in post traumatic stress disorder in F
Nemonapride	Increase plasm prolactin more in females with A1 allele than men with similar allele
Fenfluramine	Secretion of plasma cortisol response to d-fenfluramine was blunted in F but not M
Methylprednisolone	Decreased clearance in the late luteal phase. The 50% inhibitory concentration for suppression of cortisol secretion is lower in females.

	Males have more suppression of blood basophil weight.
Paroxetine	Dissociation constant for binding to platelets is lower in young F but the opposite in elderly females
Bromperidol	Plasma prolactin levels raised more in F
Growth Hormone	Larger doses required in F to achieve the same level as in M
Propoxyphine	Volume of distribution higher in M
Testosterone	Metabolism F > M
Benzylamine	Excretion 3 times greater in F following transdermal absorption
Cephradine	Slower rate of absorption and lower bioavailabilty after IM injection in F
Acetaminophen	Faster clearance in M
Terfenadine	Increased QT interval in F
Lamotrigine	Increased skin rash in F
Tegaserod	Effective for constipation predominant IBS in F but not M
Trilazad	Clearance higher in F
Methadone	Clearance higher in F
Modafinil	Clearance higher in F
Midazolam	Clearance higher in F
Nevirapine	Clearance higher in M
Ondansetron	AUC and clearance higher in F
Caffeine	Activity higher in M
Tacrine	Higher plasma levels in F
Fluvoxamine	Higher plasma levels in F
Clozapine	Higher plasma levels in F
5-Flurouracil	Clearance lower in F
Metronidazole	Clearance higher in F
DHEA	Higher plasma concentration in F
Mephobarbital	Slower metabolism in F
Insulin	M have enhanced response

Miscellaneous Facts on Toxicologic/Pharmocologic Differences in Males and Females

In females, drugs are often metabolized and eliminated differently than in males and side effects appear to be more numerous and severe. Unfortunately many drug trials exclude females.

Females are more likely to receive a drug prescription during a physician visit, to use prescription psychotropic medications and spend more money on prescription and nonprescription drugs than males.

Females are 48% more likely to use any abuseable prescription drug. Being female is a predictor of anxiolytic and narcotic analgesic use.

Adverse Drug Reaction

Females are 35% more likely to have a cutaneous drug reaction than males.

Women are 20 times more likely to develop a reaction to radiocontrast media.

Adverse reactions to antibiotics occur more often in women.

Alcohol

Alcohol has increased volume of distribution in males. Correlation curves of blood alcohol level and sedation are steeper in females.

Testosterone inhibits alcohol dehydrogenase.

Females demonstrate greater performance deficits than males when intoxicated.

Women have lower gastric glutathione-dependent formaldehyde dehydrogenase activity. This is associated with less first-pass metabolism in females.

Alcohol gastric emptying is about 40% slower in females and hepatic oxidation 10% higher in females.

Anesthesia

Women regain consciousness from anesthesia faster than men.

Neuromuscular blockade with rocuronium is more pronounced in women given the same dose (0.45mg/kg) as men.

Anticonvulsants

Phenytoin demonstrates increased clearance in the female during her luteal phase of the cycle.

Antihypertensives
>Labetalol concentrations are 80% higher in females. Gender differences in labatelol kinetics are due to differences in inactive and alpha blocking stereoisomers but not the beta-blocking stereoisomer.
>Metoprolol: females have higher concentrations given the same dose and females had greater reduction in heart rate.
>Verapamil: oral clearance is faster in men.
>Angiotensin 1 and ll infusion: The renal vasoconstrictor response to angiotensin 1 and ll is increased in females compared to men, suggesting an effect of gender on baroreflex reactivity. A negative relationship between change in heart rate and mean arterial pressure during infusion is noted only in females.
>Aspirin decreases the risk of stroke in hypertensive males.
>Diuretics tend to induce hypokalemia more commonly in females.
>ACE inhibitors induce cough more in females.

Cardiac Medications
>Digoxin for treatment of heart failure with depressed left ventricular function is associated with an increased risk of death from any cause among women but not men.

Chemotherapy
>Women tend to have more nausea and vomiting than men receiving the same agent and tend to do less well on antiemetic therapy.
>Both doxorubicin and fluorouracil show slower clearance in females.
>Both methylprednisolone and prednisolone show faster clearance in females (55% and 21% respectively).
>Women are more sensitive to the effects of methylprednisolone as demonstrated by smaller doses causing cortisol suppression in women.

Hypolipidemics
>Cerivastatin lowers LDL-C greater in females at the same dosage (At 0.4 mg dose, LDL decreased by 44% in females and 37% in males).
>The ability of fibrates to decrease triglyceride, LDL-C, and apolipoprotein levels may be greater in women.
>Plasma concentrations of lovastatin and simvastatin are higher in females by 20–50% following multiple doses.

Pain Medications
>Women experience more severe pain that lasts longer and occurs more frequently than men's pain.
>Females may have a lower pain threshold and less tolerance for pain than males.
>Women report higher pain levels for a given stimulus intensity of electrical, thermal or pressure application.
>Women may derive a greater pain benefit from kappa-opiod drugs than men. Kappa-opiods such as pentazocine, nalbuphine and butorphanol produce greater analgesia in women.
>There are gender differences in central nervous system opioid mu-receptor binding.
>Women self-prescribe and are prescribed nonsteroidal antiinflammatory agents more often than men. However among chronic NSAIAs users, men are more likely to have duodenal ulcers and erosions.
>The risk of gastric ulcers is higher in females from NSAIAs.
>Ibuprofen appears to be more effective in men in producing an analgesic response.
>Naloxone inhibits growth hormone release in females but not males.

Prescription Weight Loss Pill Usage
>Female > Male (4:1)

Psychotropic Medications
>Females take more psychotropic drugs than males.
>2/3rds of antidepressants and tranquilizers dispensed in the US are for women.
>More women take multiple medications and are more likely to have more side effects and adverse effects with psychotropic medications.
>Females have been found to have more tardive dyskinesia than men.
>Women have been found to have lower basal gastric acid secretion than men which may increase the absorption of bases such as tricyclic antidepressants, benzodiazepines and phenothiazines and decrease gastric absorption of acids such as phenytoin and barbiturates.
>Women over age 50 years are more likely than men to show neuroleptic induced agranulocytosis.
>Women with atypical depression with panic attacks respond better to MAOIs but men respond better to tricyclic antidepressants (TCAs).
>Women may need lower doses of antidepressants than men as their physiology often leads to higher serum levels of the drug.

Females more likely to respond to sertraline than imipramine while men more likely to respond to imipramine than sertraline.
Women respond to imipramine slower than men.
Premenopausal women respond better to sertraline but postmenopausal women respond similarly to imipramine and sertraline. Females are more likely to respond to paroxetine than men for treatment of depression.
Sexual side effects are reported in 60% of men and 30% of women.
Chlordiazepoxide metabolism is increased in males and its clearance decreases with age in men but not women.
Oral contraceptives decrease clearance of benzodiazepines.
Oral contraceptives increase imipramine and amitriptyline concentrations.
Women appear to respond more poorly to tricyclics than men, but respond better to selective serotonin reuptake inhibitors and monoamine oxidase inhibitors.
Platelets from men have fewer binding sites and a lower affinity for paroxetine than platelets from women.
Women are more likely to have endocrine-related adverse side effects from SSRIs than men (altered glucose metabolism, hyponatremia, and thyroid dysfunction).
Women may require lower dosages of antidepressants than men.
Women may take longer to respond to an antidepressant and require a longer course of therapy.
Estrogen may be effective for refractory depression in postmenopausal women.
Temezepam and oxazepam are benzodiazepines that are metabolized through conjugation and are cleared faster by males.
Alprazolam and diazepam are metabolized by oxidative mechanisms and are cleared faster by females.
Clearance of thiothixene is slower in females.
The rise of D1 and D2 striatal dopamine receptors parallels the early developmental appearance of motor symptoms of attention deficit hyperactivity disorder in males but not females.
The Apolipoprotein genotype response to tacrine is different in males and females. Treatment effect size was not different between epsilon 2-3 and 4 in men but was larger for epsilon 2-3 than 4 in women.

MAOIs more effective than TCAs in depressed women with panic attacks whereas TCAs more effective in depressed men with panic attacks.

The behavioral symptoms of agitation in men with Alzheimer's disease seem to respond better to resperidone than in women with AD.

The psychoactive effects of 3, 4-methylenedioxymethamphetamine (MDMA) are more intense in females, especially perceptual changes, thought disturbances, and fear of loss of body control.

Pulmonary Medications

Use of glucocorticosteroids to treat asthma and cystic fibrosis has been shown to cause more growth suppression in boys than in girls, especially when used prepubertally.

Theophylline shows changes in clearance, half-life and peak concentrations during the menstrual cycle. The half-life lengthens from 5.4 to 7.8 hours from the ovulatory to the luteal phase due to decreased clearance.

Females are more sensitive to the hypokalemic, chronotropic and electrocardiographic sequelae of inhaled terbutaline.

Thrombolytic Therapy

Females seem to have more intracranial bleeding from thrombolytics used to treat acute MIs.

Tobacco

Nicotine replacement therapy is less effective in females and women have more difficulty quitting smoking.

Women that smoke appear 1–3 times more likely to develop oral cancer. The interaction of smoking and alcohol consumption increases the risk more than 5 times for oral cancer in women.

Gender Differences in Susceptibility to Environmental Exposures

Women with lung cancer are more likely to have GC-TA mutations than men. Also women have higher carcinogen adduct formation and more of their tumors contain c-erb-2 staining than men.

Aflatoxin

Liver cancer: M > F (2.5–5 times)

Arsenic

Females appear more likely to develop bladder and kidney cancer.

Benzene
> T1/2: F > M
>
> Women have a higher blood/air partition coefficient, longer half-life and higher maximum velocity of metabolism for benzene than men. This results in women metabolizing 23–26% more benzene than men when exposed to the same scenario.

Dioxin
> Plasma dioxin concentrations have been found to be elevated in women as compared to men exposed to the same level.
>
> Females exposed to dioxin appear to produce a lower male to female birth ratio than normal.
>
> Dioxin-related Cancer
>> Men: Leukemia, esophageal, rectal
>> Female: Liver, stomach, colon
>> Hodgkin's Disease: Women > Men

Lead
> Hematologic changes (FEP, ALA): F > M

Ozone
> Ozone affects female and male runners differently, and female runners are impacted differently depending on their menstrual cycle stage.

Pesticide Exposure
> Non-Hodgkin's Lymphoma: Men > Women
> Soft tissue Sarcoma: Men > Women

Tobacco-related Cancers
> Odds ratios for cancer
>> Lung (bronchogenic): Females 8.1, Male 4.6
>> Oral: Female 5.0, Male 2.0

Trichloroethylene
> Acid Metabolite: F > M
> Alcohol Metabolite: M > F

Other/Miscellaneous

Animal Bites
    Male > Female
    Males are more likely to be bitten by dogs; females are more likely to be bitten by cats.

Arterial Gas Embolism
    Male > Female

Asbestosis
    Male > Female

Birth Asphyxia and Other Respiratory Conditions
    Male > Female (1.6:1)

Birth Weight
    Males are heavier at birth than females on average.

Blunt Trauma
    Males older than 45 years have a higher incidence of pneumonia; however females with pneumonia have about 3–5 times higher risk of death than males after blunt trauma.

Building-Related Illness, Nonspecific Symptoms
    Female > Male

Burns
    Male > Female (2:1)

Cancer Mortality
    Males > Female
    The rate in 1994 was 253.2 per 100,000 men and 165.7 per 100,000 women.

Congenital Anomalies
    Male > Female (1.7:1)

Decompression Sickness
Male > Female
95% of cases occur in males.

Dieting
On any given day in the US, over 50 million females and 24 million males say they are on a diet.

Disability
Female > Male
The prevalence rate of disability in 1999 was 24% in females and 20% in males.
Males reported higher disability for heart trouble/hardening of arteries, deafness/hearing problems.
Elderly women require assistance with activities of daily living more than elderly men.
Women report more arthritis/rheumatism.

Drowning
Male > Female (10:1)

Falls in Older Adults
Female > Male

Fetal Movements
Males display more leg movements per minute during antenatal and postnatal development.

Fractures of Skull or Face
Male > Female (3.2:1)

Healthcare Utilization
Females receive more health services than men but are less satisfied with their health care.

Hiccups
Male > Female (4:1)

Homicide
Male > Female

Injury
Male > Female (2:1)
Males appear to engage in more risky behaviors, and to be supervised less by someone that may protect them from these risks.

Males more likely to have the following injuries:

Injury	% Male
Motor Vehicle	68
Drowning	80
Fire	60
Ingestion of object	54
Firearm	87
Poison by solid/liquid	76
Poison by gas	74

Leading Causes of Death by Gender for All Age Groups

	Male	*Female*
#1	Heart Disease	Heart Disease
#2	Cancer	Cancer
#3	Cerebrovascular	Cerebrovascular Disease
#4	Accidents	Chronic Obstructive Pulmonary Disease
#5	COPD	Pneumonia/Influenza
#6	Pneumonia/Influenza	Diabetes Mellitus
#7	Diabetes Mellitus	Accidents
#8	Suicide	Alzheimer's Disease
#9	Cirrhosis of Liver	Nephritis
#10	Homicide	Septicemia

Left Handers
  Male > Female

Life Expectancy
  Female > Male
  In 1996 the life expectancy for females was 6.4 years longer than males.

Marathon Running Hyponatremia
  Females > Males
  Females are also more symptomatic.

Measles, Mumps, Rubella Vaccine Reaction
  Female > Male
  The relative risk of fever and rash was 2.35 in females and 1.36 in males.

Mosquito Bites
  Males are more readily bitten than females.

Motor Vehicle Crashes
Male drivers experience 3.5 fatal wrecks per 100 million miles vs. 2.2 fatal wrecks for women. However female drivers involved in 2.3 nonfatal injury crashes per million vehicle miles traveled compared to 1.8 for male drivers.
Males are more likely to speed and account for 68% of traffic fatalities. Males also drive more miles per year than females.
Women drink and drive less frequently than men and are involved in fewer alcohol-related crashes.
Males are more likely to take risk while driving and sensation seeking. Females arrested for drinking and driving are more likely to be coming from a friend's home while males more likely to be coming from a bar.

Multiple Chemical Sensitivity
Female > Male (7:1)

Near Drowning
Males > Females

Occupational Upper Extremity Musculoskeletal Complaints
Female > Male

Ocular Chemical Burn
Male > Female

Open Wounds and Injuries to Blood Vessels
Male > Female (3:1)

Orthopedic Visits
> 70% of office visits by men but only 55% by women are injury related.
Young men and old females are the groups most likely to visit an orthopedist.
Knee problems #1 reason for visit by both sexes.
Women are more likely to seek care for feet, ankle, hip and wrist problems and sensation disorders.
Men are more likely to seek care for back, shoulder and elbow problems.
Women are more likely to be diagnosed by orthopedist with carpal tunnel syndrome, synovitis/tenosynovitis or other rheumatic illnesses.
Men are more likely to be diagnosed with knee dislocations, intervertebral discs disorders and hand/finger fractures.

Athletic injuries that females are at higher risk for include stress fractures and injuries of the shoulder, knee, back and pelvis.

Physical Activity
  Males > Females
  Males are more likely to get physical activity throughout the year.

Placenta Previa
  The male: female ratio at birth is higher in women with placenta previa than in those without (1.19:1.05).

Premature births
  The prevalence of handicaps is 3 times higher in males that survive. Premature born boys have been found to have higher incidence of asthma, intellectual disability, and higher mortality.
  Survival after perinatal asphyxia is greater in females.

Pressure Ulcer
  Female > Male
  Due to survival difference, majority occur in the elderly.

Radiocontrast Media Reaction
  Female > Male (20:1)

Rectal Temperature
  Newborn males have a lower rectal temperature than newborn females during the first 5 days of life (37.068 vs. 37.168 degrees C).

Sedentary Americans
  Females > Males
  31.5% vs. 27.9%

Snake Bites
  Male > Female

Sprain, Strain
  Male > Female

Thermal Tolerance
  Female ability to thermoregulate in hot, humid conditions, may be better than males due to lower sweat production rates in females which slows dehydration.
  Females have higher skin temperatures in moderate or severe heat stress suggesting a higher skin blood flow.

However females do not tolerate cold environments as well possibly because of greater surface area to mass ratio of females even at the same level of fatness.

Females have a larger surface area-to-mass ratio than men.

In dry, severe heat where air temperature is higher than skin temperature, women will gain heat faster by convection and have a smaller mass to store it in which results in increased core temperature.

In humid areas women have an advantage over males because of their greater surface area to mass ratio allowing for more evaporation.

When air temperature is below skin temperature, women lose heat faster than men through radiation and convection.

Women are less thermally sensitive to cold water. In cold water, women cool more rapidly than men at rest but there is not a greater metabolic response by women.

Men may be more metabolically sensitive to cold air stress. Men respond to cold air with bradycardia and increased stroke volume, while women show no change in these parameters.

Tobacco Use

Male > Female

Men tend to smoke to reduce boredom and fatigue, and to improve concentration.

Women tend to smoke to reduce stress and control weight.

Men respond more strongly to nicotine's analgesic and stimulation effects. Men are more successful in quitting smoking compared to women. Women tend to respond better to behavior modification coupled with social support in smoking cessation efforts. Additionally women respond better to bupropion and clonidine than to nicotine replacement therapy.

Passive smoking may be more harmful for boys. In boys the risk of adult wheezing increases by 15–30% respectively if one or both parents smoke whereas the same not seen in girls.

A study has shown that men that smoked > 20 years are 3.3 times more at risk for developing lung cancer than those that smoked less than 20 years, and the corresponding risk for women is 2.7. After 40 years of smoking, the risk ratio is 4 for men and 3.3 for women. Women are 1.2–1.7 times higher risk for all types of lung cancer for the same level of cigarette smoke exposure as men.

Risk of lung cancer from exposure to environmental tobacco smoke (second-hand smoke) is higher in males.

Females that smoke are twice as likely to develop diabetes as men.

Females have more difficulty quitting smoking and cite hunger as a symptom of withdrawal more than men.

Women may be more susceptible to effects of smoking on pulmonary function.

Smoking may be a stronger risk factor for heart attacks in women.

Training and Sports Injuries

Female > Male

Probably due to low physical fitness and body composition (higher percent body fat in female).

In a study of Army trainees, females experienced twice as many injuries.

Transplants

Liver transplants are less successful when donated by a female, especially when the recipient is male.

Cardiac transplants appear more successful in males.

Female heart transplants have more significant rejection episodes than male recipients at both 3 and 12 months after the transplant. In addition female heart transplant recipients tend to require additional maintenance steroids to control rejection.

Transplants appear more successful with same-gender donors.

References

Books

American Psychiatric Association: Diagnostic and Statistical Manual of Mental Disorders, Fourth Edition. Washington, DC, American Psychiatric Association, 1994.

Ballenger JJ, Snow JB Jr. ed. Otorhinolaryngology: Head and Neck Surgery, Fifteenth Edition. Media, Pennsylvania, Williams and Wilkins, 1996.

Baum GL, Celli BR, Crapo JD, Karlinsky JB, ed. Textbook of Pulmonary Diseases, Sixth Edition, Volume 1. Philadelphia, Pennsylvania, Lippincott-Raven Publishers, 1997.

Braunwald E, Zipes DP, Libby P, ed. Heart Disease: A Textbook of Cardiovascular Medicine, Sixth Edition, Volume 1. Philadelphia, Pennsylvania, WB Saunders Company, 2001.

Brenner BM, ed. Brenner and Rector's The Kidney, Sixth Edition, Volume 1. Philadelphia, Pennsylvania, WB Saunders Company, 2000.

Dambro MR, ed. Griffith's Five-Minute Clinical Consult 2000. Philadelphia, Pennsylvania, Lippincott Williams and Wilkins, 2000.

Feldman M, Scharschmidt BF, Sleisenger MH, ed. Sleisenger and Fordtran's Gastrointestinal and Liver Disease: Pathophysiology/Diagnosis/Management, Sixth Edition, Volume 1. Philadelphia, Pennsylvania, WB Saunders Company, 1997.

Ferri FF, ed. Ferri's Clinical Advisor: Instant Diagnosis and Treatment. St. Louis, Missouri, Mosby, 2000.

Fitzpatrick TB, Johnson RA, Wolff K, Suurmond D. Color Atlas and Synopsis of Clinical Dermatology: Common and Serious Diseases. New York, New York, McGraw-Hill, 2001.

Freedberg IM, Eisen AZ, Wolff K, Austen KF, Goldsmith LA, Katz SE, Fitzpatrick TB, Ed. Fitzpatrick's Dermatology in General Medicine, Fifth Edition. New York, New York, McGraw-Hill, 1993.

Hupp JR, Williams TP, Vallerand WP. The Five-Minute Clinical Consult for Dental Professionals. Baltimore, Maryland, Williams and Wilkins, 1996.

Julian DG, Wenger NK, ed. Women and Heart Disease. St. Louis, Missouri, Mosby, 1997.

Kane KS, Ryder JB, Johnson RA, Baden HP, Stratigos A. Color Atlas and Synopsis of Pediatric Dermatology. New York, New York, McGraw-Hill, 2002.

Klippel JH, Weyand CM, Wortmann RL, ed. Primer On The Rheumatic Diseases, Eleventh Edition. Atlanta, Georgia, 1997.

Lee GR, Foerster J, et. al, ed. Wintrobe's Clinical Hematology, Tenth Edition, Volume 1. Baltimore, Maryland, Williams and Wilkins, 1998.

Lemcke DP, Pattison J, Marshall LA, Cowley DS, ed. Primary Care of Women. Norwalk, Connecticut, Appleton and Lange, 1995.

Lenter C, ed. Geigy Scientific Tables, 8th revision. Basle, Switzerland. Ciba-Geigy, Ltd. 1981.

Middleton E Jr., Ellis EF, Yunginger JW, et. al., ed. Allergy Principles and Practice, Volume 1. St. Louis, Missouri, Mosby, 1998.

Miles A. Women, Health and Medicine. Bristol, Pennsylvania, Open University Press, 1991.

Nelson, Leonard B, ed., Harley's Pediatric Ophthalmology, Fourth Edition. Philadelphia, Pennsylvania, W.B. Saunders Company, 1991.

Ness RB, Kuller LH, ed. Health and Disease Among Women: Biological and Environmental Influences. New York, New York, Oxford University Press, Inc., 1999.

Newell FW. Ophthalmology Principles and Concepts, Eighth Edition. St. Louis, Missouri, Mosby-Year Book, Inc, 1996.

Ruddy S, Harris ED Jr., Sledge CB, ed. Kelley's Textbook of Rheumatology, Sixth Edition. Philadelphia, Pennsylvania, WB Saunders Company, 2001.

Salvendy G. Handbook of Human Factors and Ergonomics, 2nd Edition. New York, NY, John Wiley and Sons, Inc., 1997.

Setlow VP, Lawson CE, Wood NF, ed. Gender Differences in Susceptibility to Environmental Factors: A Priority Assessment. Institute of Medicine. Washington D.C., National Academy Press, 1998.

Townsend CM, Beauchamp RD, Evers BM, Mattox KL, ed. Sabiston Textbook of Surgery: The Biological Basis of Modern Surgical Practice, Sixteenth Edition. Philadelphia, Pennsylvania, W.B. Saunders Company, 2001.

Victor M, Ropper AH. Adams and Victor's Principles of Neurology, Seventh Edition. New York, New York, McGraw-Hill, 2001.

Warwick R, Williams PL, ed. Gray's Anatomy, Thirty-fifth Edition. Philadelphia, Pennsylvania, W.B. Saunders Company, 1973.

Wilson JD, Foster DW, Kronenerg HM, Larsen PR, ed. Williams Textbook of Endocrinology, Ninth Edition. Philadelphia, Pennsylvania, WB Saunders Company, 1998.

Wizemann TM, Pardue ML, eds. Committee on Understanding the Biology of Sex and Gender Differences. Exploring the Biological Contributions to Human Health: Does Sex Matter? Board on Health Sciences Policy. Institute of Medicine. Washington, D.C., National Academy Press, 2001.

Journals

Acharya DU, Heber ME, Dore CJ, et al. Ambulatory intraarterial blood pressure in essential hypertension: Effects of age, sex, race, and body mass-the Northwick Park Hospital Database study. Am J Hypertens 1996; 31:943–952.

Adams KF, Vincent LM, McAllister SM, el-Ashmawy H, Sheps DS. The influence of age and gender on left ventricular response to supine exercise in asymptomatic normal subjects. Am Heart J 1987; 113(3):732–742.

Adeeb N, Ton SH, Muslim N. Effect of age, weight, race and sex on blood pressure and erythrocyte sodium pump characteristics. Clin Exp Hypertens A 1990; 12(6):1115–1134.

Agarwal J. Women had a lower risk than men for mortality after coronary revascularization. ACP Journal Club 1999; 130:49.

Ahmed SA, Hissong B D, Verthelyi D, Donner K, Becker K, Karpuzoglu-Sahin E. Gender and risk of autoimmune diseases: Possible role of estrogenic compounds. Environmental Health Perspectives 1999; 107(Suppl 5):681–686.

Airewele GE, Sigurdson Aj, Wiley KJ, Frieden BE, Caldarera LW, Riccardi VM, Lewis RA, Chintogumpala MM, Ater JL, Plon SE, Bondy ML. Neoplasms in neurofibromatosis 1 are related to gender but not to family history of cancer. Genet Epidemiol 2001; 20(1):75–86.

Aitken ML, Franklin JL, Pierson DJ, Schoene RB. Influence of body size and gender on control of ventilation. J Appl Physiol 1986; 60(6):1894–1899.

Allen LS, Richey MF, Chai YM, Gorski RA. Sex differences in the corpus callosum of the living human being. J Neurosci 1991; 11(4):933–942.

Allen MY, Higginbotham EJ. Impact of hormonal changes on the eye. The Female Patient 2000; 25:57–60.

Almli CR, Ball RH, Wheeler ME. Human fetal and neonatal movement patterns: Gender differences and fetal-to-neonatal continuity. Dev Psychobiol 2001; 38(4):252–273.

American Cancer Society, Inc. 2000.Cancer statistics 2000. CA-A Cancer Journal for Clinicians. 2000; 50(1).

Anastos K, Gange SJ, Lau B, Weiser B, Detels R, Giorgi JV, Margolick JB, Cohen M, Phair J, Melnick S, Rinaldo CR, Kovacs A, Levine A, Landesman S, Young M, Munoz A, Greenblatt RM. Association of race and gender with HIV-1 RNA levels and immunologic progression. J Acquir Immune Defic Syndr 2000; 24(3):218–226.

Anderson AE. Gender-related aspects of eating disorders: A Guide to Practice. J Gend Specif Med 1999; 2(1):47–54.

Anderson GD. Sex differences in drug metabolism: Cytochrome P-450 and uridine diphosphate glucuronosyltransferase. J Gend Specif Med 2002; 5(1):25–33.

Angele MK, Schwacha MG, Ayala A, Chaudry IH. Effect of gender and sex hormones on immune responses following shock. Shock 2000; 14(2):81–90.

Anonymous. Ankylosing spondylitis: Is susceptibility determined by female sex? Women's Health Orthopedic Edition 2000; 3(2):49.
Anonymous. Exercise and oxygen uptake in women with high blood pressure. Women's Health Orthopedic Edition 1999; 2(5):26.
Anonymous. Long-term evolution of CRMO. Women's Health Orthopedic Edition 2000; 3(2):72.
Antman K, Chang Y. Kaposi's sarcoma. N Engl J Med 2000; 342(14):1027–1038.
Arandt EA. Gender differences in musculoskeletal health. J Gend Specif Med 2000; Special Issue:58–64.
Armellini F, Zamboni M, Bosello O. Hormones and body composition in humans: Clinical studies. Int J Obes Relat Metab Disord 2000; 24(Suppl 2):S18–S21.
Aronson D, Burger AJ. Gender-related differences in modulation of heart rate in patients with congestive heart failure. J Cardiovasc Electrophysiol 2000; 11(10):1071–1077.
Ashley MJ. Smoking and diseases of the gastrointestinal system: An epidemiological review with special reference to sex differences. Can J Gastroenterol 1997; 11(4):345–352.
Atroshi I, Gummesson C, Johnsson R, Ornstein E, Ranstam J, Rosen I. Prevalence of carpal tunnel syndrome in a general population. JAMA 1999; 282(2):153–158.
Aurigemma GP, Gaasch WH. Gender differences in older patients with pressure-overload hypertrophy of the left ventricle. Cardiology 1995; 86(4):310–317.
Ayanian JZ. Increased mortality among middle-aged women after myocardial infarction: Searching for mechanisms and solutions. Ann Intern Med 2001; 134(3):239–241.
Aydintug AO, Domenech I, Cervera R, Khamashta MA, Jedryka-Goral A, Vianna JL, Hughes GR. Systemic lupus erythematosus in males: Analysis of clinical and laboratory features. Lupus 1992; 1(5):295–298.
Aytug N, Giral A, Imeryuz N, enc FY, Bekiroglu N, Aktas G, Ulusoy NB. Gender influence on jejungal migrating motor complex. Am J Physiol Gastrointest Liver Physiol 2001; 280(2):G255–263.
Bailar JC III, Gornik HL. Cancer undefeated. N Engl J Med 1997; 336(22):1569–1574.
Bakx JC, van den Hoogen HJ, van den Bosch WJ, et al. Development of blood pressure and the incidence of hypertension in men and women over an 18-year period: Results of the Nijmegen Cohort Study. J Clin Epidemiol 1999; 52:531–538.
Barakat K, et al. Acute myocardial infarction in women: Contribution of treatment variable to adverse outcome. American Heart Journal 2000; 140:740–746.
Baraona E, Abittan CS, Dobmen K, Moretti M, Pozzato G, Chayes ZW, Schaefer C, Lieber CS. Gender differences in pharmacokinetics of alcohol. Alcohol Clin Exp Res 2001; 25(4):502–507.
Barbarino A, De Marinis L, Mancini A, D'Amico C, Passeri M, Zuppi P, Sambo P, Tofani A. Sex-related naloxone influence on growth hormone-re-

leasing hormone-induced growth hormone secretion in normal subjects. Metabolism 1987; 36(2):105–109.

Barone GW, Moursi MM, Eidt JF. Aortoiliac vascular disease in younger women. The Female Patient 1998; 23:27–35.

Barr WB, Jaffe J, Wassrestein J, Michelson WJ, Stein BM. Regional distribution of cerebral arteriovenous malformations: Interactions with sex and handedness. Arch Neurol 1989; 46(4):410–412.

Barrett AM. Probable alzheimer's disease: Gender-related issues. J Gend Specif Med 1999; 2(1):55–60.

Beim GM. Sports Injuries in Women. Women's Health Orthopedic Edition 1999; 2(1):27–34.

Belay ED, Bresee JS, Holman RC, Khan AS, Shahriari A, Schonberger LB. Reye's syndrome in the United States from 1981 through 1997. N Engl J Med 1999; 340(18):1377–1382.

Bell NS, Mangione TW, Hemenway D, Amoroso PJ, Jones BH. High injury rates among female army trainees—a function of gender? Am J Prev Med 2000; 18(3S):141–146.

Benetos A. Sex influences mortality risk associated with diastolic blood pressure. J Am Coll Cardiol 2001; 37:163–168.

Bengtsson S, Berglund H, Gulyas B, Cohen E, Savic I. Brain activation during odor perception in males and females. Neuroreport 2001; 12(9):2027–2033.

Berg MJ. Drugs, vitamins and gender. J Gend Specif Med 1998; http://www.mmhc.com/jgsm/articles/JGSM9809/Berg.html.

Berg MJ. Drugs, vitamins, and gender. J Gend Specif Med 1999; http://www.mmhc.com/jgsm/articles/JGSM9902/pharmfocjan.html.

Berg MJ. Gender-specific prescribing: Medications and the menstrual cycle. J Gend Specif Med 1998; http://www.mmhc.com/jgsm/articles/JGSM9812/pharmfoc.html.

Berg MJ. Pharmacokinetics and pharmacodynamics of cardiovascular agents. J Gend Specif Med 1999; http://www.mmhc.com/jgsm/articles/JGSM9908/pharm.html.

Berhane K, McConnell R, Gilliland F, Islam T, Gauderman WJ, Avol E, London SJ, Rappaport E, Margolis HG, Peters JM. Sex-specific effects of asthma on pulmonary function in children. Am J Respir Crit Care Med 2000; 162(5):1723–1730.

Bidoggia H, Maciel JP, Capalozza N, Mosca S, Blaksley EJ, Valverde E, Bertran G, Arini P, Biagetti MO, Quinteiro RA. Sex differences on the electrocardiographic pattern of cardiac repolarization: Possible role of testosterone. Am Heart J 2000; 140(24):678–683.

Bilbao JR, Rica L, Vazquez JA, Busturia MA, Castano L. Influences of sex and age at onset on autoantibodies against insulin, GAD65 and IA2 in recent onset type 1 diabetic patients. Horm Res 2000; 54(4):181–185.

Bilezikian J. Gender specificity and osteoporosis. J Gend Specif Med 2000; 3(7):6–12.

Bilger RC, Matthies ML, Hammel DR, Demorest ME. Genetic implications of gender differences in the prevalence of spontaneous otoacoustic emissions. J Speech Hear Res 1990; 33(3):418–432.

Bishop KM, Wahlsten D. Sex differences in the human corpus callosum: Myth or reality? Neurosci Biobehav Rev 1997; 21(5):581–601.

Bjornson C L, Mitchell I. Gender differences in asthma in childhood and adolescence. J Gend Specif Med 2000; 3(8):57–61.

Boling EP. Gender and osteoporosis: Similarities and sex-specific differences. J Gend Specif Med 2001; 4(2):36–43.

Bowman DM, Brown DK, Kimberley BP. An examination of gender differences in DPOAE phase delay measurements in normal-hearing human adults. Hear Res 2000; 142(1–2):1–11.

Bradley CS, Singh GS. Interstitial cystitis. The Female Patient 2000; 25:81.

Bradley KA, Badrinath S, Bush K, Boyd-Wickizer J, Anawalt B. Medical risks for women who drink alcohol. J Gen Intern Med Sep 1998; 13:627–639.

Branch DR. Antiarrhythmic drugs pose higher risk in women. Family Practice News May 1 1997:40–41.

Branch DR. Smoking cessation, withdrawal worse at menstrual cycle's end. Family Practice News Apr 15 1997:38.

Breslau N, Chilcoat H, Schultz LR. Anxiety disorders and the emergence of sex differences in major depression. J Gend Specif Med 1998; 1(3):33–39.

Breslau N. Gender differences in trauma and posttraumatic stress disorder. J Gend Specif Med 2002; 5(1):34–40.

Brooks LJ, Strohl KP. Size and mechanical properties of the pharynx in healthy men and women. Am Rev Respir Dis 1992; 146(6):1394–1397.

Brown EA, Shelley ML, Fisher JW. A pharmacokinetic study of occupational and environmental benzene exposure with regard to gender. Risk Analysis 1998; 18(2):205–213.

Bulaj ZJ, Ajioka RS, Phillip JD, LaSalle BA, Jorde LB, Griffen LM, Edwards CQ, Kushner JP. Disease related conditions in relatives of patients with hemochromatosis. N Engl J Med 2000; 343(21):1529–1535.

Bulaj ZJ, Griffen LM, Jorde LB, Edwards CQ, Kushner JP. Clinical and biochemical abnormalities in people heterozygous for hemochromatosis. N Engl J Med 1996; 335(24):1799–1805.

Buschang PH, Tanguay R, Demirjian A, La Palme L, Goldstein H. Sexual dimorphism in mandibular growth of French-Canadian children 6 to 10 years of age. Am J Phys Anthropol 1986; 71(1):33–37.

Buskila D, Neumann L, Alhoashle A, Abu-Shakra M. Fibromyalgia syndrome in men. Semin Arthritis Rheum 2000; 30(1):47–51.

Cahil L, Haier RJ, White NS, Fallon J, Kilpatrick L, Lawrence C, Potkin SG, Alkire MT. Sex-related differences in amygdala activity during emotionally influenced memory storage. Neurobiol Learn Mem 2001; 75(1):1–9.

Calam J, Springer CJ, Bojarski JC, Francis-Reme ML. Postprandial gastrin concentration are higher in female patients with duodenal ulcers. Digestion 1989; 42(3):163–166.

Cali RL, Blatchford GJ, Perry RE, Pitsch RM, Thorson AG, Christensen MA. Normal variation in anorectal manometry. Dis Colon Rectum 1992; 35(12):1161–1164.

Calle-Rodrigue RDP, Giannini C, Scheithauer BW, Lloyd RV, Wollan PC, Kovacs KT, Stefaneanu L, Ebright AB, Abboud CF, Davis DH. Prolactinomas in male and female patients: A comparative clinicopathologic study. Mayo Clin Proc 1998; 73:1046–1052.

Calvo MS, Eastell R, Offord KP, Bergstralh EJ, Burritt MF. Circadian variation in ionized calcium and intact parathyroid hormone: Evidence for sex differences in calcium homeostasis. J Clin Endocrinol Metab 1991; 72(1):69–76.

Campaigne BN, Wishner KL. Gender-specific health care in diabetes mellitus. J Gend Specif Med 2000; 3(1):51–58.

Campbell WW, Ostlund RE Jr, Joseph LJ, Farrell PA, Evans WJ. Relationships of plasma C-peptide and gender to the urinary excretion of inositols in older people. Horm Metab Res 2001; 33(1):44–51.

Camper-Kirby D, Welch S, Walker A, Shiraishi I, Setchell KD, Schaefer E, Kajstura J, Anversa P, Sussman MA. Myocardial Akt activation and gender: Increased nuclear activity in females versus males. Circ Res 2001; 88(10):1020–1027.

Cankar K, Finderle Z, Strucl M. Gender differences in cutaneous laser doppler flow response to local direct and contralateral cooling. J Vasc Res 2000; 37(3):183–188.

Canto JG, Shlipak MG, Rogers WJ, Malmgren JA, Frederick PD, Lambrew CT, Ornato JP, Barron HV, Kiefe CI. Prevalence, clinical characteristics, and mortality among patients with myocardial infarction presenting without chest pain. JAMA 2000; 283(24):3223–3229.

Caplan LR. Diagnosis and treatment of ischemic stroke. JAMA 1991; 266(17):2413–2418.

Cassidy JW, Ditty KM. Gender differences among newborns on a transient otoacoustic emissions test for hearing. J Music Ther 2001; 38(1):28–35.

Castelao JE, Yuan JM, Skipper PL, Tannenbaum SR, Gago-Dominquez M, Crowder JS, Ross RK, Yu MC. Gender-and smoking-related bladder cancer risk. J Natl Cancer Inst 2001; 93(7):538–545.

Catlin A, Brophy S, Blake D. Impact of sex on inheritance of ankylosing spondylitis: A cohort study. Lancet 1999; 354:1687–1690.

Catlin EA, Powell SM, Manganaro TF, Hudson PL, Ragin RC, Epstein J, Donahoe PK. Sex-specific fetal lung development and mullerian inhibiting substance. Am Rev Respir Dis 1990; 141(2):466–476.

CDC. 1997. Demographic differences in notifiable infectious diseases morbidity-United States, 1992–1994. MMWR 1997; 46(28):638–640.

CDC. 1997. Mortality patterns-preliminary data, United States, 1996. MMWR 1997; 46(40):941–944.

CDC. 1997. State and sex-specific prevalence of selected characteristics-behavioral risk factor surveillance system, 1994 and 1995. MMWR 1997; 46(No. SS-3).

CDC. 1997. Youth risk behavior surveillance, National College Health Risk Behavior Survey-United States, 1995. MMWR 1997; 46(No. SS-6).

CDC. 1998. Changes in mortality from heart failure-United States, 1980–1995. MMWR 1998; 47(30):633–637.

CDC. 1998. Prevalence and impact of chronic joint symptoms-seven states, 1996. MMWR 1998; 47(17):345–350.

CDC. 1999. Youth risk behavior surveillance—National Alternative High School Youth Risk Behavior Survey, United States 1998; MMWR 1999; 48(No. SS-7).

CDC. 2000. State-and sex-specific prevalence of selected characteristics-behavioral risk factor surveillances system, 1996 and 1997. MMWR 2000; 49(No. SS-6).

CDC. 2001. Primary and secondary syphilis-United States, 1999. MMWR 2001; 50(7):113–116.

CDC. Chronic liver disease. MMWR 1993; 41(Nos. 52-53).

CDC. Mortality from coronary heart disease and acute myocardial infarction-United States, 1998. MMWR 2001; 50(6):90–93.

Celesia GG, Kaufman D, Cone S. Effects of age and sex on pattern electroretinograms and visual evoked potentials. Electroencephalogr Clin Neurophysiol 1987; 68(3):161–171.

Celius EG, Harbo HF, Egeland T, Vartdal F, Vandvik B, Spurkiand A. Sex and age at diagnosis are correlated with the HLA-DR2, DQ6 haplotype in multiple sclerosis. J Neurol Sci 2000; 178(2):132–135.

Center JR, Nguyen TV, Schneider D, Sambrook PN, Eisman JA. Mortality after all major types of osteoporotic fracture in men and women: An observational study. Lancet 1999; 353:878–882.

Chafin CC, Tolley EA, George CM, demirkan K, Kuhl DA, Pugazhenthi M, Self TH. Gender differences in metered-dose inhaler-spacer device technique. Pharmacotherapy 2000; 20(11):1324–1327.

Chandra NC, et al. Observations of the treatment of women in the United States with myocardial infarction: A report from the National Registry of Myocardial Infarction. Arch Intern Med 1998; 158:981–988.

Cheng H, Rogers JD, Sweany AE, Dobrinska MR, Stein EA, Tate AC, Amin RD, Quan H. Influence of age and gender on the plasma profiles of 3-hydroxy-3-methylglutaryl-coenzyme A (HMG-CoA) reductase inhibitory activity following multiple doses of lovastatin and simvastatin. Pharm Res 1992; 9(12):1629–1633.

Chow RS, Medri MK, Martin DC, Leekam RN, Agur AM, McKee NH. Sonographic studies of human soleus and gastrocnemius muscle architecture: Gender variability. Eur J Appl Physiol 2000; 82(3):236–44.

Chow WH, Devesa SS, Warren JL, Fraumeni JF Jr. Rising incidence of renal cell cancer in the United States. JAMA 1999; 281(17):1628–1631.

Clapp R, Ozonoff D. Where the boys aren't: Dioxin and the sex ratio. Lancet, 2000; 355:1838–1839.

Clauw DJ, Groner KH. Fibromyalgia. The Female Patient 2000; 25:61.

Clouse WD, Hallett JW, Schaff HV, Gayari MM, Ilstrup DM, Melton LJ III. Improved prognosis of thoracic aortic aneurysms. JAMA 1998; 280(22):1926–1929.

Collazos J, Mayo J, Martinez E, Blanco M. Muscle infections caused by salmonella species: Case report and review. Clinical Infectious Diseases 1999; 29:673–677.

Colliander EB, Tesch PA. Bilateral eccentric and concentric torque of quadriceps and hamstring muscles in females and males. Eur J Appl Physiol Occup Physiol 1989; 59(3):227–232.

Comston A, Coles A. Multiple sclerosis. Lancet 2002; 359:1221–1231.

Cooke JP, Creager MA, Osmundson PJ, Shepherd JT. Sex differences in control of cutaneous blood flow. Circulation 1990; 82(5):1607–1615.

Cowell CT, Briody J, Lloyd-Jones S, Smith C, Moore B, Howman-Giles R. Fat distribution in children and adolescents—the influence of sex and hormones. Hormone Res 1997; 48(Suppl 5):93–100.

Crabtree TD, Pelletier SJ, Gleason TG, Pruett TL, Sawyer RG. Gender-dependent differences in outcome after the treatment of infection in hospitalized patients. JAMA 1999; 282(22):2143–2148.

Crandall C. Gender differences in osteoporosis treatment: A review of clinical research. J Gend Specif Med 2000; 3(8):42–46.

Cruickshanks KJ, et al. Prevalence of hearing loss in older adults in Beaver Dam, Wisconsin: The epidemiology of hearing loss study. Am J Epidemiol 1998; 148:879–886.

Cureton K, Bishop P, Hutchinson P. Sex difference in maximal oxygen uptake. Effect of equating hemoglobin concentration. Eur J Appl Physiol 1986; 54:656–60.

Dao TT, LeResche L. Gender differences in pain. J Orofac Pain 2000; 4(3):169–184.

DaSilva JA. Sex hormones and glucocorticoids: Interactions with the immune system. Ann NY Acad Sci 1999; 876:102–117.

Davis DL, Gottlieb M, Stampnitzky J. Reduced ratio of male to female births in several industrial countries. JAMA 1998; 279(13):1018–1023.

Davis PB. The gender gap in cystic fibrosis survival. J Gend Specif Med 1999; 2(2):47–51.

Davis SN, Shavers C, Costa F. Gender-related differences in counterregulatory responses to antecedent hypoglycemia in normal humans. J Clin Endocrinol Metab 2000; 85(6):2145–2157.

De Bellis MD, Keshavan MS, Beers SR, Hall J, Frustaci K, Masalehdan A, Noll J, Boring AM. Sex differences in brain maturation during childhood and adolescence. Cereb Cortex 2001; 11(6):552–557.

De Groen PC, Gores GJ, LaRusso NF, Gunderson LL, Nagorney DM. Biliary tract cancers. N Engl J Med 1999; 341(18):1368–1378.

de Zwart BC, Frings-Dresen MH, Kilbom A. Gender differences in upper extremity musculoskeletal complaints in the working population. Int Arch Occup Environ Health 2001; 74(1):21–30.

Demir M, Acarturk E. Clinical characteristics influence aortic root dimension and blood flow velocity in healthy subjects. Angiology 2001; 52(7):457–461.

Demissie K, Breckenridge MB, Joseph L, Rhoads GG. Placenta previa: Preponderance of male sex at birth. Am J Epidemiol 1999; 149(9):824–830.

Digre KB, Corbett JJ. Pseudotumor cerebri in men. Arch Neurol 1988; 45(8):866–872; Erratum in: Arch Neurol 1989; 46(2):172.

Dimitrow PP, Czarnecka D, Strojny JA, Kawecka-Jaszcz K, Dubiel JS. Impact of gender on the left ventricular cavity size and contractility in patients with hypertrophic cardiomyopathy. Int J Cardiol 2001; 77(1):43–48.

Diwan VK, Thorson A. Sex, gender and tuberculosis. Lancet 1999; 353:1000–1001.

Dodge JT Jr, Brown BG, Bolson EL, Dodge HT. Lumen diameter of normal human coronary arteries. Influence of age, sex, anatomic variation, and left ventricular hypertrophy or dilation. Circulation 1992; 86(1):232–246.

Donegan WL. Cancer of the male breast. J Gend Specif Med 2000; 3(4):55–58.

Donnellan CA. Motor neuron disease (amyotrophic lateral sclerosis) in the elderly. Clinical Geriatrics 1997; 5(11):31.

Doraiswamy PM, Potts JM, Axelson DA, Husain MM, Lurie SN, Na C, Escalona PR, McDonald WM, Figiel GS, Ellinwood EH Jr. et al. MR assessment of pituitary gland morphology in healthy volunteers: Age- and gender-related differences. Am J Neuroradiol 1992; 13(5):1295–1299.

Dresler CM, Fratelli C, Babb J, Everley L, Evans AA, Clapper ML. Gender differences in genetic susceptibility for lung cancer. Lung Cancer 2000; 30(3):153–160.

Drewnowski A, Kristal A, Cohen J. Genetic taste responses to 6-n-propylthiouracil among adults: A screening tool for epidemiological studies. Chem Senses 2001; 26(5):483–489.

Durrant JD, Sabo DL, Hyre RJ. Gender, head size, and ABR's examined in large clinical sample. Ear Hear 1990; 11(3):210–214.

Egger HL, Angold A, Costello EJ. Headaches and psychopathology in children and adolescents. J Am Acad Child Adolesc Psychiatry 1998; 37:951–958.

Elands J, van Woudenberg A, Resink A, de Kloet ER. Vasopressin receptor capacity of human blood peripheral mononuclear cells is sex dependent. Brain Behav Immun 1990; 4(1):30–38.

Elia J, Ambrosini PJ, Rapoport JL. Treatment of attention-deficit-hyperactivity disorder. N Engl J Med 1999; 340(10):780–788.

Elsaleh H, Joseph D, Grieu F, Zeps N, Spry N, Iacopetta B. Association of tumour site and sex with survival benefit from adjuvant chemotherapy in colorectal cancer. Lancet 2000; 355:1745–1750.

Endicott J. Gender similarities and differences in the course of depression; J Genc Specif Med 1998; 1(3):40–43.

Escalona PR, McDonald WM, Doraiswamy PM, Boyko OB, Husain MM, Figiel GS, Laskowitz D, Ellinwood EH Jr, Krisnan KR. In vivo stereological assessment of human cerebellar volume: Effects of gender and age. Am J Neuroradiol 1991; 12(5):927–929.

Fagot-Campagna A, Saaddine J, Venkat Narayan KM, Goldschmid M. Re. Sex differences in risk factors for clinical diabetes mellitus in a general population: A 12-year follow-up of the Finnmark Study. Am J Epidemiol 1999; 149(11):1073–1074.

Feifel D. Attention-deficit hyperactivity disorder in adults. Postgraduate Medicine 1996; 100(3):207–211, 215–218.

Feliciani C, Amerio P. Madelung's disease: Inherited from an ancient Mediterranean population? N Engl J Med 1999; 340(19):1481.

Fernandez-Sola J, Nicolas-Arfelis JM. Gender differences in alcoholic cardiomyopathy. J Gend Specif Med 2002; 5(1):41–47.

Finotti P, Piccoli A, Carraro P. Alteration of plasma proteinase-antiproteinase system in type 1 diabetic patients. Influence of sex and relationship with metabolic control. Diabetes Res Clin Pract 1992; 18(1):35–42.

Fletcher CV, Acosta EP, Strykowski JM. Gender differences in human pharmacokinetics and pharmacodynamics. J Adolesc Health 1994; 15(8):619–629.

Forastiere A, Koch W, Trotti A, Sidransky D. Head and neck cancer. N Engl J Med 2001; 345(26):1890–1898.

Frank E, Thase ME, Spanier CA, Reynolds CF III, Kupfer DJ. Gender-specific response to depression treatment. J Gend Specif Med 1999; 2(4):40–44.

Frankhauser MP. Psychiatric disorders in women: Psychopharmacologic treatments. J Am Pharm Assoc (Wash) 1997; NS37(6):667–678.

Freedman RR, Sabharwal SC, Desai N. Sex differences in peripheral vascular adrenergic receptors. Circ Res 1987; 61(4):581–585.

Freeman HP, Payne RP. Racial injustice in health care. N Engl J Med 2000; 342(14):1045–1046.

Fried SK, Kral JG. Sex differences in regional distribution of fat cell size and lipoprotein lipase activity in morbidly obese patients. Int J Obes 1987; 11(2):129–140.

Frisch M, Hjalgrim H, Jaeger AB, Biggar RJ. Changing patterns of tonsillar squamous cell carcinoma in the United States. Cancer Causes and Control 2000; 11:489–495.

Fulco CS, Rock PB, Muza SR, Lammi E, Braun B, Cymerman A, Moore LG, Lewis SF. Gender alters impact of hypobaric hypoxia on adductor pollicis muscle performance. J App Physiol 2001; 91(1):100–108.

Fuller AK, LeRoy JB. Personality disorders: An overview for the physician. Southern Medical Journal 1993; 86(4):430–436.

Gale EA, Gillespie KM. Diabetes and gender. Diabetologia 2001; 44(1):3–15.

Gariepy J, Denarie N, Chironi G, Salomon J, Levenson J, Simon A. Gender differences in the influence of smoking on arterial wall thickness. Atherosclerosis 2000; 153(1):139–145.

Gary A. Gender differences in the prevalence of metabolic complications in familial partial lipodystrophy (dunnigan variety). J Clin Endocrinol Metab 2000; 85(5):1776–1782.

Genecov JS, Sinclair PM, Dechow PC. Development of the nose and soft tissue profile. Angle Orthod 1990; 60(3):191–198.

George JN. Idiopathic thrombocytopenic purpura. The Female Patient 2000; 25:66.

Gesensway D. Reasons for sex-specific and gender-specific study of health topics. Ann Intern Med 2001; 135(10):935–938.

Giordana SH, Buzdar AU, Hortobagyi GN. Breast cancer in men. Ann Intern Med 2002; 137 (8):678–687.

Giron-Gonzalez JA, Moral FJ, Elvira J, Garcia-Gil D, Guerrero F, Gavilan I, Escobar L. Consistent production of a higher TH1:TH2 cytokine ratio by stimulated T cells in men compared with women. Eur J Endocrinol 2000; 143(1):31–36.

Gladman DD, Brubacher B, Buskila D, Langevitz P, Farewell VT. Psoriatic spondyloarthropathy in men and women: A clinical, radiographic, and HLA study. Clin Invest Med 1992; 15(4):371–375.

Glass AG, Hoover RN; The emerging epidemic of melanoma and squamous cell skin cancer. JAMA 1989; 262(15):2097–2100.

Goldstein JM, Santangelo SL, Simpson JC, Tsuang MT. The role of gender in identifying subtypes of schizophrenia; a latent class analytic approach. Schizophr Bull 1990; 16(2):263–275.

Gonzalez-Gay MA, Rodriguez-Valverda V, Blanco R, Fernandez-Sueiro J, Armona J, Figueroa M, Martinez-Taboada V. Polymyalgia rheumatica without significantly increased erythrocyte sedimentation rate: A More Benign Syndrome. Arch Intern Med 1997; 157:317–320.

Goto T, Klyce SD, Zheng X, Maeda N, Kuroda T, Ide C. Gender-and age-related differences in corneal topography. Cornea 2001; 20(3):270–276.

Grachev ID, Apkarian AV. Chemical heterogeneity of the living human brain: A proton MR spectroscopy study on the effects of sex, age, and brain region. Neuroimage 2000; 11(5 Pt 1):554–563.

Grachev ID, Apkarian AV. Chemical mapping of anxiety in the brain of healthy humans: An in vivo 1H-MRS study on the effects of sex, age, and brain region. Hum Brain Mapp 2000; 11(4):261–272.

Graff J, Brinch K, Madsen JL. Gastrointestinal mean transit times in young and middle-aged healthy subjects. Clin Physiol 2001; 21(2):253–259.

Graham TE. Thermal, metabolic, and cardiovascular changes in men and women during cold stress. Med Sci Sports Exerc 1988; 20(5 Suppl):S185–S192.

Greenblatt DJ, Friedman H, Burstein ES, Scavone JM, Blyden GT, Ochs HR, Miller LG, Harmatz JS, Shader RI. Trazodone kinetics: Effect of age, gender and obesity. Clin Pharmacol Ther 1987; 42(2):193–200.

Greenlee RT, Hill-Harmon MB, Murray T, Thun M. Cancer statistics, 2001; CA-Cancer J Clin 2001; 51(1):15–36.

Grisso JA, Battistini M, Ryan L. Women's health textbooks: Codifying science and calling for change. Ann Intern Med 1998; 129(11):916–918.

Groen PC, Gores G, LaRusso N, Gunderson L, Nagorney D. Biliary tract cancer. N Eng J Med 2001; 341 (18); 1368–1378.

Gur RC, Mozley PD, Resnick SM, Gottlieb GL, Kohn M, Zimmerman R, Herman G, Atlas S, Grossman R, Berretta D, et al. Gender differences in age effect on brain atrophy measured by magnetic resonance imaging. Proc Natl Acad Sci USA 1991; 88(7):2845–2849.

Gur RE, Gur RC. Gender differences in regional cerebral blood flow. Schizophr Bull 1990; 16(2):247–254.

Haasbeek JF. Adolescent idiopathic scoliosis. Postgraduate Medicine 1997; 101(6):207–209, 215–216.

Hadler NM. Knee pain is the malady—not osteoarthritis. Ann Intern Med 1992; 116(7):598–599.

Haffner SM, Valdez R, Morales PA, Mitchell BD, Hazuda HP, Stern MP. Greater effect of glycemia on incidence of hypertension in women than in men. Diabetes Care 1992; 15(10):1277–1284.

Hain TC, et al. Mal de Debarquement. Archives of Otolaryngology-Head & Neck Surgery 1999; 125:615–620.

Hales D. Finally, Better treatment for women (And men too). Parade Magazine Mar 7 1999:10–12.

Hammond CJ, Ophth FR, Sneider H, Spector TD, Gilbert CE. Genetic and environmental factors in age-related nuclear cataracts in monozygotic and dizygotic twins. N Eng J Med 2000; 342 (24):1786–1790.

Hanley PC, Zinsmeister AR, Clements IP, Bove AA, Brown ML, Gibbons RJ. Gender-related differences in cardiac response to supine exercise assessed by radionuclide angiography. J Am Coll Cardiol 1989; 13(3):624–629.

Harik-Khan RI, Wise RA, Fleg JL. The effect of gender on the relationship between body fat distribution and lung function. J Clin Epidemiol 2001; 54(4):399–406.

Harrington RD, Hooton TM. Urinary tract infection risk factors and gender. J Gend Specif Med 2000; 3(8):27–34.

Harris A, et al. Aging affects the retrobulbar circulation differently in women and men. Archives of Ophthalmology 2000; 118:1076–1080.

Haut JS, Beckwith BE, Petros TV, Russell S. Gender differences in retrieval from long-term memory following acute intoxication with ethanol. Physiol Behav 1989; 45(6):1161–1165.

Hawker GA, Wright JG, Coyte PC, Williams JI, Harvey B, Glazier R, Badley EM. Differences between men and women in the rate of use of hip and knee arthroplasty. N Engl J Med 2000; 342(14):1016–1022.

Hayes SN, Taler SJ. Hypertension in women: Current understanding of gender differences. Mayo Clinic Proc 1998; 73:157–165.

Haymart MR, Allen J, Blumenthal RS. Optimal management of dyslipidemia in women and men. J Gend Specif Med 1999; 2(6):37–42.

Hayward CS, Kalnins WV, Kelly RP. Gender-related differences in left ventricular chamber function. Cardiovasc Res 2001; 49(2):340–350.

Heintze U, Birkhed D, Bjorn H. Secretion rate and buffer effect of resting and stimulated whole saliva as a function of age and sex. Swed Dent J 1983; 7(6):227–238.

Hinojosa-Laborde C, Chapa I, Lange D, Haywood JR. Gender differences in sympathetic nervous system regulation. Clin Exp Pharmacol Physiol 1999; 26(2):122–126.

Hofman MA, Swaab DF. Sexual dimorphism of the human brain: Myth and reality. Exp Clin Endocrinol 1991; 98(2):161–170.

Holloway JB, Baechle TR. Strength training for female athletes. A review of selected aspects. Sports Med 1990; 9(4):216–228.

Horowitz SH, Krarup C. Conduction studies of the normal sural nerve. Muscle Nerve 1992; 15(3):374–383.

Horvath E, Kovacs K. Gonadotroph adenomas of the human pituitary: Sex-related fine structural dichotomy. A histologic, immunocytochemical, and electron-microscopic study of 30 tumors. Am J Pathol 1984; 117(3):429–440.

Hoyert DL, Rosenberg HM. 1999. Mortality from Alzheimer's Disease: An Update. National Vital Statistics Report:Centers for Disease Control and Prevention 1999; 47(20).

Hoyt L. HIV infection in women and children. Postgraduate Medicine 1997; 102(4):165–166,169–171,176.

Hugues CJ, Asmar RG, London GM, Safar ME. Age- and sex-related changes in the ratio between ankle and brachial systolic pressure in normal subjects. Angiology 1988; 39(3 Pt 1):219–226.

Humphries KH, Kerr CR, Connolly SJ, et al. New-onset atrial fibrillaition. Sex differences in presentation, treatment, and outcome. Circulation 2001; 103:2365–2370.

Huston LJ, Wojytys EM. Neuromuscular performance characteristics in elite female athletes. AJSM 1998; 24:427–435.

Imperiale TF, Wagner DR, Lin CY, Larkin GN, Rogge JD, Ransohoff DF. Risk of advanced proximal neoplasms in asymptomatic adults according to the distal colorectal findings. N Engl J Med 2000; 343(3):169–174.

Iribarren C, Sidney S, Sternfeld B, Browner WS. Calcification of the aortic arch risk factors and association with coronary heart disease, stroke, and peripheral vascular disease. JAMA 2000; 283(21):2810–2815.

Ishunina TA, Salehi A, Swaab DF. Sex- and age-related P75 neurotrophin receptor expression in the human supraoptic nucleus. Neuroendocrinology 2000; 71(4):243–251.

Jacobs AK, Kelsey SF, Brooks MM, et al. Better outcome for women compared with men undergoing coronary revasculaarization. A report from the Bypass Angioplasty Revascularization Investigation (BARI).Circulation.1998; 98:1279–1285.

Jacobs G, Costa F, Shannon JR, Robertson RM, Wathen M, Stein M, Biaggioni I, Ertl A, Black B, Robertson D. The neuropathic postural tachycardia syndrome. N Engl J Med 2000; 343(14):1008–1014.

James GD, Sealey JE, Muller F, Alderman M, Madhavan S, Laragh JH. Renin relationship to sex, race and age in a normotensive population. J Hypertens Suppl 1986; 4(5):S387–S389.

Jancin B. Second ca afflicts women survivors more than men. Family Practice News May 15 1997; 27(10):1,4.

Johansson AG. Gender differences in growth hormone response in adults. J Endocrinol Invest 1999; 22(5 Suppl):58–60.

Johnson CC, Peterson EL, Ownby DR. Gender differences in total and allergen-specific Immunoglobulin E (IgE) concentrations in a population-based cohort from birth to age four years. Am J Epidemiol 1998; 147(12):1145–1152.

Johnson JA, Akers WS, Herring VL, Wolfe MS, Sullivan JM. Gender differences in labetalol kinetics: Importance of determining stereoisomer kinetics for racemic drugs. Pharmacotherapy; 20(6):622–628.

Jones FS. Are men's and women's brains different? NCMJ 1998; 59(3):191–192.

Jones G, Glisson M, Hynes K, Cicuttini F. Sex and site differences in cartilage development: A possible explanation for variations in knee osteoarthritis in later life. Arthritis Rheum 2000; 43(11):2543–2549.

Jorgensen MJ, Marras WS, Granata KP, Wiand JW. MRI-derived moment-arms of the female and male spine loading muscles. Clin Biomech (Bristol, Avon) 2001; 16(3):182–193.

Joyner JM, Hutley LJ, Cameron DP. Glucocorticoid receptors in human preadipocytes: Regional and gender differences. J Endocrinol 2000; 166(1):145–152.

Kaawach W, Ecklund K, Di Canzio J, Zurakowski D, Waters PM. Normal ranges of scapholunate distance in children 6 to 14 years old. J Pediatr Orthop 2001; 21(4):464–467.

Kalaria VG, Zareba W, Moss AJ, Pancio G, Marder VJ, Morrissey JH, Weiss HJ, Sparks CE, Grenberg H, DwyerE, Goldstein R, Watelet LF. Gender-related differences in thrombogenic factors predicting recurrent cardiac events in patients after acute myocardial infarction. The THROMBO Investigators. Am J Cardiol 2000; 85(12):1401–1408.

Kane S. Caring for women with inflammatory bowel disease. J Gend Specif Med 2001; 4(1):54–59.

Kannus P, Parkkari J, Koshinen S, Niemi S, Palvanen M, Jarvinen M, Vuori I. Fall-induced injuries and deaths among older adults. JAMA 1999; 281(20):1895–1899.

Kansaku K, Yamaura A, Kitazawa S. Sex differences in lateralization revealed in the posterior language areas. Cereb Cortex 2000; 10(9):866–872.

Karlstadt RG. Gender-based biology and the gastrointestinal tract. J Gend Specif Med 2000; Special Issue:41–52.

Kaufman LD, Heinicke MH, Hamburger M, Gorevic PD. Male lupus: Prevalence of IgA deficiency, 7S IgM and abnormalities of reticuloendothelial system Fc-receptor function. Clin Exp Rheumatol 1991; 9(3):265–269.

Kauhanen J. Review: Some health risks associated with drinking alcohol are greater for women than for men. ACP Journal Club 1999:50.

Kaur V, Gum D. Tropical diseases and women. Clinics in Dermatology 1997; 15:171–177.

Kearney-Cooke A. Gender differences and self-esteem. J Gend Specif Med 1999; 2(3):46–52.

Kendler KS, Thornton LM, Prescott CA. Gender differences in the rates of exposure to stressful life events and sensitivity to their depressogenic effects. Am J Psychiatry 2001; 158(4):587–593.

Kendler KS. Gender differences in the genetic epidemiology of major depression. J Gend Specif Med 1998; 1(2):28–31.

Khan LK, Serdula MK, Bowman BA, Williamson DF. Use of prescription weight loss pills among U.S. adults in 1996–1998. Ann Intern Med 2001; 134(4):282–286.

Kiely DK, et al. Identifying nursing home residents at risk for falling. J Amer Geriatrics Soc 1998; 46:551–555.

Kiser AC, Roberts CS. Spontaneous hemopneumothorax in women. Southern Medical Journal 2000; 93(12):1209–1211.

Kiss A, Meryn S. Effect of sex and gender on psychosocial aspects of prostate and breast cancer. BMJ 2001; 323(3):1055–1058.

Kneale BJ, Chowienczyk PJ, Brett SE, Coltart DJ, Ritter JM. Gender differences in sensitivity to adrenergic agonists of forearm resistance vasculature. J Am Coll Cardiol 2000; 36(4):1233–1238.

Koh SC, Yuen R, Viegas OA, Chua SE, Ng BL, Sen DK, Ratnam SS. Plasminogen activators t-PA, u-PA and its inhibitor (PAI) in normal males and females. Thromb Haemost 1991; 66(5):581–585.

Kojouri K, Vesley SK, George JN. Quinine-associated thrombotic thrombocytopenic purpura-hemolytic uremic syndrom: Frequency, clinical features, and long-term outcomes. Ann Intern Med 2001; 135(12):1047–1051.

Konradi C, Kornhuber J, Sofic E, Heckers S, Riederer P, Beckmann H. Variations of monamines and their metabolites in the human brain putamen. Brain Res 1992; 579(2):285–290.

Kratz A, Lewandrowski KB. Normal reference laboratory values. N Engl J Med 1998; 339(15):1063–1072.

Krivickas LS, Suh D, Wilkins J, Hughes VA, Roubenoff R, Frontera WR. Age- and gender-related differences in maximum shortening velocity of skeletal muscle fibers. Am J Phys Med Rehabil 2001; 80(6):447–457.

Krogstad BS, Dahl BL, Eckersberg T, Ogaard B. Sex differences in signs and symptoms from masticatory and other muscles in 19-year-old individuals. J Oral Rehabil 1992; 19(5):435–440.

Kuruvilla A, Peedicayil J, Srikrishna G, Kuruvilla K, Kanagasabapathy AS. A study of serum prolactin levels in schizophrenia: Comparison of males and females. Clin Exp Pharmacol Physiol 1992; 19(9):603–606.

La Rue A. Gender differences in mood and cognition; in estrogen and mental illness in aging. Presentations in FocusTM 1997:4–6.

Labiche LA, Chan W, Saldin KR, Morgenstern LB. Sex and acute stroke presentation. Ann Emerg Med 2002; 40(5):453–460.

Lackner TE, Cloyd JC, Thomas LW, et al. Antiepileptic drug use in nursing home residents: Effect of age, gender, and comedication on patterns of use. Epilepsia 1998; 39(10):1083–1087.

Lahita RG. Gender and the immune system. J Gend Specif Med Oct 2000; 3(7):19–22.

Lai HC, FitzSimmons SC, Allen DB, Kosorok MR, Rosenstein BJ, Campbell PW, Farrell PM. Risk of persistent growth impairment after alternate-day prednisone treatment in children with cystic fibrosis. N Engl J Med 2000; 342(12):851–859.

Lai Z, Roos P, Olsson Y, Larsson C, Nyberg F. Characterization of prolactin receptors in human choroids plexus. Neuroendocrinology 1992; 56(2):225–233.

Lambe EK. Dyslexia, gender, and brain imaging. Neuropsycologia 1999; 37(5):521–536.

Langenberg AG, Corey L, Ashley R, Leong W, Straus S, A prospective study of new infections with herpes simplex virus Type 1 and Type 2. Chiron HSV Vaccine Study Group. N Engl J Med 1999; 341:1432–1438.

Larkin M. Sex differences in lung-cancer susceptibility explained? Lancet 2000; 355:121.

Laughlin GA, Barrett-Connor E. Sexual dimorphism in the influence of advanced aging on adrenal hormone levels: The Rancho Bernardo Study. Clin Endocrinol Metab 2000; 85(10):3561–3568.

Laumann EO, Paik A, Rosen RC. Sexual dysfunction in the United States. JAMA 1999; 281(6):537–544.

Lazarus GM. Gender-specific medicine in pediatrics. J Gend Specif Med 2001; 4(1):50–53.

Legato MJ. Gender and the Heart: Sex-specific differences in normal anatomy and physiology. J Gend Specif Med 2000; 3(4):22, 25–26.

Leiblum SR. Sexual problems and dysfunction: Epidemiology, classification, and risk factors. J Gend Specif Med 1999; 2(5):41–45.

Leveille SG, Guralnik JM, Ferrucci L, Hirsch R, Simonsick E, Hochberg MC. Foot pain and disability in older women. Am J Epidemiol 1998; 148(7):657–665.

Levine AM. Evaluation and management of HIV-infected women. Ann Intern Med 2002; 136(3):228–242.

Levy D, Kenchaiah S, Larson MG, Benjamin EJ, Kupka MJ, Ho KK, Murabito J, Vasan RS. Long-term trends in the incidence of and survival with heart failure. N Eng J Med 2002; 347(18):1397–1402.

Liechti ME, Gamma A, Vollenweider FX. Gender differences in the subjective effects of MDMA. Psychopharmacology (Berl) 2001; 154(2):161–168.

Lindman R, Eriksson A, Thornell LE. Fiber type composition of the human female trapezius muscle; enzyme-histochemical characteristics. Am J Anat 1991; 190(4):385–392.

Lloyd-Jones DM, Larson AG, Beiser A, Levy D. Lifetime risk of developing coronary heart disease. Lancet 1999; 353:89–92.

Lockshin MD. Antiphospholipid antibody. JAMA 1997; 277(19):1549–1551.

Lockshin MD. Rheumatoid arthritis in 2000. The Female Patient 2000; 25:78–80.

Lowe NJ. Managing acne in adult women. Patient Care 1997; 31:30–43.

Luukinen H, et al. Prognosis of diastolic and systolic orthostatic hypotension in older persons. Arch Intern Med 1999; 159:273–280.

MacMillan HL, Fleming JE, Trocme N, Boyle MH, Wong M, Racine YA, Beardslee WR, Offord DR. Prevalence of child physical and sexual abuse in the community. JAMA 1997; 278(2):131–135.

Mahmoud SF. Lawrence-Seip Syndrome: Report of a case from Egypt. Cutis 1997; 60:91–93.

Maisel WH, Rawn JD, Stevenson WG. Atrial fibrillation after cardiac surgery. Ann Intern Med 2001; 135(12):1061–1073.

Majetschak M, Christensen B, Obertacke U, Waydhas C, Schindler AE, Nast-Kolb D, Schade FU. Sex differences in posttraumatic cytokine release of endotoxin-stimulated whole blood: Relationship to the development of severe sepsis. J Trauma 2000; 48(5):832–838.

Makkar RR, Fromm BS, Steinman RT, Meissner MD, Lehmann MH. Female gender as a risk factor for Torsades do Pointes associated with cardioascular drugs. JAMA 1993; 270(21):2590–2597.

Malamitsi-Puchner A, Tziotis J, Tsonou A, Protonotariou E, Sarandakou A, Creatsas G. Changes in serum levels of vascular endothelial growth factor in males and females throughout life. J Soc Gynecol Investig 2000; 7(5):309–312.

Mallon WJ, Brown HR, Nunley JA. Digital ranges of motion: Normal values in young adults. J Hand Surg [Am] 1991; 16(5):882–887.

Mallory KJ, Bahinski A. Cardiovascular disease and arrhythmias: Unique risks in women. J Gend Specif Med 1999; 2(1):37–44.

Marcus DA. Gender differences in chronic headache in a treatment-seeking population. J Gend Specif Med 2000; 3(6):50–53.

Marcus DA. Management of headache in women. J Gend Specif Med 1999; 2(4):47–50.

Mark DB. Sex Bias in cardiovascular care. JAMA 2000; 283(5):659–661.

Marras WS, Jorgensen MJ, Granata KP, Wiand B. Female and male trunk geometry: Size and predicition of the spine loading trunk muscles derived from MRI. Clin Biomech (Bristol, Avon) 200; 16(1):38–46.

Marrugat J, Sala J, Masia R, Pavesi M, Sanz G, Valle V, Molina L, Seres L, Elosua R. Mortality differences between men and women following first myocardial infarction. JAMA 1998; 280(16):1405–1409.

Marugo M, Torre G, Bernasconi D, Fazzuoli L, Cassulo S, Giordano G. Androgen receptors in normal and pathological thyroids. Endocrinol Invest 1991; 14(1):31–35.

Massie DL, Green PE, Campbell KL. Crash involvement rates by driver gender and the role of average annual mileage. Accid Anal and Prev; 29(5):675–685.

Mayer EA, Naliboff B, Lee O, Munakata J, Chang L. Review article: Gender-related differences in functional gastrointestinal disorders. Aliment Pharmacol Ther 1999; 13 (Supp 2):65–69.

Mazhar AR, Johnson RJ, Gillen D, Stivelman JC, Ryan MJ, Davis CL, Stehman-Breen, CO. Risk factors and mortality associated with calciphylaxis in end-stage renal disease. Kidney Int 2001; 60(1):324–332.

McFadden D. A speculation about the parallel ear asymmetries and sex differences in hearing sensitivity and otoacoustic emissions. Hear Res 1993; 68(2):143–151.

McMaster ML, Goldstein AM, Bromley CM, Ishibe N, Parry DM. Chordoma: Incidence and survival patterns in the United States, 1973–1995. Cancer Causes and Control 2001; 12:1–11.

Mehilli J, Kastrati A, Dirschinger J, Bollwein H, Neumann FJ, Schomig A. Differences in prognostic factors and outcomes between women and men undergoing coronary artery stenting. JAMA 2000; 284(14):1799–1805.

Meier-Kriesche HU, Ojo AO, Leavey SF, Hanson JA, Leichtman AB, Magee JC, Cibrik DM, Kaplan B. Gender differences in the risk for chronic renal allograft failure. Transplantation 2001; 71(3):429–432.

Meisinger C, Thorand B, Schneider A, Stieber J, Doring A, Lowel H. Sex differences in risk factors for incident Type 2 diabetes mellitus, The MONICA Augsburg Cohort Study. Arch Intern Med 2000; 162:82–89.

Mercurio MG. Gender-specific medicines and dermatology: Clinical implications. J Gend Specif Med 2000; 3(7):23–28.

Mercurio MG, Gogstetter DS. Androgen physiology and the cutaneous pilosebaceous unit. J Gend Specif Med 2000; 3(4):59–64.

Mercurio MG. Gender and dermatology. J Gend Specif Med 1998; 1(1):16–20.

Meryn S, Jadad A. The future of men and their health. BMJ 2001; 323(3):1013–1014.

Messerli FH, Garavaglia GE, Schmieder RE, Sundgaard-Riise K, Nanez BD, Amodeo C. Disparate cardiovascular findings in men and women with essential hypertension. Ann Intern Med 1987; 107(2):158–161.

Messing K, Dumais L, Romito P. Prostitutes and chiney sweeps both have problems: Towards full integration of both sexes in the study of occupational health. Soc Sci Med 1993; 36(1):47–55.

Michelena HI, Ezekowitz MD. Atrial Fibrillation: Are there gender differences? J Gend Specif Med 2000; 3(6):44–49.

Miglior S, Brigatti L, Velati P, Balestreri C, Rossetti L, Bujtar E, Orzalesi N. Relationship between morphometric optic disc parameters, sex and axial length. Curr Eye Res 1994; 13(2):119–124.

Mii S, Nakamura K, Takeo K, Kurimoto S. Analysis of human tear proteins by two-dimensional electrophoresis. Electrophoresis 1992; 13(6):379–382.

Milano G, Etienne MC, Cassuto-Viguier E, Thyss A, Santini J, Frenay M, Renee N, Schneider M, Demard F. Influence of sex and age on fluorouracil clearance. J Clin Oncol 1992; 10(7):1171–1175.

Millstein RA. Gender and drug abuse research. J Gend Specif Med 1998; 1(3):44–47.

Mitchell LA, Zhang T, Tingle AJ. Differetial antibody responses to rubella virus infection in males and females. J Infect Dis 1992; 166(6):1258–1265.

Mobley DF, Baum N. Interstitial cystitis. Postgraduate Medicine 1996; 99(5):201–204, 207–208, 214.

Mohri M, et al. Angina pectoris caused by coronary microvascular spasm. Lancet 1998; 351:1165–1169.

Mokdad AH, Serdula MK, Dietz WH, Bowman BA, Marks JS, Koplan JP. The spread of the obesity epidemic in the United States, 1991–1998. JAMA 1999; 282(16):1519–1522.

Moore AL, Mocroft A, Madge S, Devereux H, Wilson D, Phillips AN, Johnson M. Gender differences in virologic response to treatment in an HIV-positive population: A cohort study. J Acquir Immune Defic Syndr 2001; 26(2):159–163.

Moore-Sledge, CM. Evaluation and management of first seizures in adults. American Family Physician 1997; 56(4):1113–1120.

Morley JE. Nutrition and the older female: A review. J Am Coll Nutr 1993; 12(4):337–343.

Mortensen EL, Hogh P. A gender difference in the association between APOE genotype and age-related cognitive decline. Neurology 2001; 57(1):89–95.

Nagy E, Loveland KA, Orvos H, Molnar P. Gender-related physiologic differences in human neonates and the greater vulnerability of males to developmental brain disorders. J Gend Specif Med 2001; 4(1):41–49.

Nagy E. Gender-related differences in rectal temperature in human neonates. Early Hum Dev 2001; 64(1):37–43.

Napier K. Sex differences are "biologically relevant" in neurologic disorders. Primary Care Neurology Reviews 1997; 1:12–13.

Napolitano LM, Greco ME, Rodriguez A, Kufera JA, West RS, Scalea TM. Gender differences in adverse outcomes after blunt trauma. J Trauma 2001; 50(2):274–280.

Netzer NC, Stoohs RA, Netzer CM, Clark K, Strohl KP. Using the Berlin questionnaire to identify patients at risk for the sleep apnea syndrome. Ann of Intern Med 1999; 131(7):485–491.

Newman AB, Arnold AM, Burke GL, O'Leary DH, Manolio TA. Cardiovascular disease and mortality in older adults with small abdominal aortic

aneurysms detected by ultrasonography: The cardiovascular health study. Ann Intern Med 2001; 134:182–190.
Niedfelt MW, Young CC. Common foot problems in women. The Female Patient 1998; 23:15–32.
Nies AS, Andros EA, Gerber JG. Platelet alpha 2-adrenergic receptor responsiveness is increased in elderly men but not in elderly women. Clin Pharmacol Ther 1992; 52(6):605–608.
Nunn AJ, Gregg I. New regression equations for predicting peak expiratory flow in adults. BMJ 1998; 298:1068–1070.
Nyberg F, et al. Environmental tobacco smoke and lung cancer in nonsmokers: Does time since exposure play a role? Epidemiology 1998; 9:301–308.
O'Connor C, Thornley KS, Hanly PJ. Gender differences in the polysomnographic features of obstructive sleep apnea. Am J Respir Crit Care Med 2000; 161(5):1465–1472.
Oberholzer A, Keel M, Zellweger R, Steckholzer U, Trentz D, Ertel W. Incidence of septic complications and multiple organ failure in severely injured patients is sex specific. J Trauma 2000; 48(5):932–937.
Oberman AS, Wei JY. Older women and heart disease. The Female Patient 1998; 23:10–13.
Okiishi CG, Paradiso S, Robinson RG. Gender differences in depression associated with neurologic illness: Clinical correlates and pharmacologic response. J Gend Specif Med 2001; 4(2):65–72.
Olmos JM, Amado JA, Riancho JA, Albajar M, Gonzalez-Macias J. Sex and age distribution of 1,25(OH) 2D3 receptors in peripheral blood mononuclear cells from normal human subjects. Bone 1990; 11(6):407–409.
Ose L, Luurila O, Eriksson J, Olsson A, Lithell H, Widgren B. Cerivastatin gender effect: Sub-analyses of results from a multinational, randomized, double-blind study. Current Medical Research and Opinion 2000; 16(2):80–87.
Ostmeier H, Schumann J, Otto F, Krieg V, Fuchs B, Biess B, Burg G, Suter L. The relationship between characteristics of the tumor cells and sex of the patients in primary malignant melanomas. J Cancer Res Clin Oncol 1991; 117(4):364–366.
Ott BR, Heindel WC, Tan Z, Noto RB. Lateralized cortical perfusion in women with Alzheimer's disease. J Gend Specif Med 2000; 3(6):29–35.
Pansarasa O, Castagna L, Colombi B, Vecchiet J, Felzani G, Marzatico F. Age and sex differences in human skeletal muscle: Role of reactive oxygen species. Free Radic Res 2000; 33(3):287–293.
Parilo MA, Gonzales CL. Acute quadriplegia in a 34-year-old man. Southern Medical Journal 2000; 93(12):1221–1223.
Paula FJ, Pimenta WP, Saad MJ, Paccola GM, Piccinato CE, Foss MC. Sex-related differences in peripheral glucose metabolism in normal subjects. Diabete Metab 1990; 16(3):234–239.
Peck S, Peck L. Selected aspects of the art and science of facial esthetics. Semin Orthod 1995; 1(2):105–126.

Perry TL, Ohde RN, Ashmead DH. The acoustic bases for gender identification from children's voices. J Acoust Soc Am 2001; 109(6):2988–2998.
Persky V, Ostrow D, Langenberg P, Ruby E, Bresolin L, Stamler J. Hypertension and sodium transport in 390 healthy adults in Chicago. J Hypertens 1990; 8(2):121–128.
Petri M. 2000. Systemic lupus erythematosus: Women's health issues. Bull Rheum Dis 2000; 49(8):1–3.
Pido-Lopez J, Imami N, Aspinall R. Both age and gender affect thymic output: More recent thymic migrants in females than males as they age. Clin Exp Immunol 2001; 125(3):409–413.
Pillar G, Malhotra A, Fogel R, Beauregard J, Schnall R, White DP. Airway mechanics and ventilation in response to resistive loading during sleep: Influence of gender. Am J Respir Crit Care Med 2000; 162(5):1627–1632.
Pinto S, Coppo M, Paniccia R, Prisco D, Gori AM, Attanasio M, Abbate R. Sex related differences in platelet TxA2 generation. Prostaglandins Leukot Essent Fatty Acids 1990; 40(3):217–221.
Pitzalis MV, Iacoviello M, Masari F, Guida P, Romito R, Forleo C, Vulpis V, Rizzon P. Influence of gender and family history of hypertension on autonomic control of heart rate, diastolic function and brain natriuretic peptide. J Hypertens 2001; 19(1):143–148.
Poduval RD, Bananian S, Rajiv D, Kumar KS, Fomberstein B. Systemic lupus erythematosus in males: A retrospective study with a review of the literature. J Gend Specif Med 2000; 3(5):29–32.
Pointer JS. Evidence that a gender difference in intraocular pressure is present from childhood. Opthalmic Physiol Opt 2000; 20(2):131–136.
Pope M, Ashley MJ, Ferrence R. The carcinogenic and toxic effects of tobacco smoke: Are women paticularly susceptible? J Gend Specif Med 1999; 2(6):45–51.
Rahman AR, McDevitt DG, Struthers AD, Lipworth BJ. Sex differences in hypokalaemic and electrocardiographic effects of inhaled terbutaline. Thorax 1992; 47(12):1056–1059.
Rathore SS, Wang Y, Krumholz HM. Sex-based differences in the effect of digoxin for the treatment of heart failure. N Eng J Med 2002; 347(18); 1403–1411.
Raz N, Torres IJ, Acker JD. Age, gender, and hemispheric differences in human striatum: A quantitative review and new data from in vivo MRI morphometry. Neurobiol Learn Mem 1995; 63(2):133–142.
Reid RL, Quigley ME, Yen SSC. Pituitary apoplexy: A review. Arch Neurol 1985; 42:712–719.
Relling MV, Lin JS, Ayers GD, Evans WE. Racial and gender differences in N-acetyltransferase, xanthine oxidase, and CYP1A2 activities. Clin Pharmacol Ther 1992; 52(6):643–658.
Remoue F, To Van D, Schacht AM, Picquet M, Garraud O, Vercruysse J, Ly A, Capron A, Riveau G. Gender-dependent specific immune response during chronic human Schistosomiasis haematobia. Clin Exp Immunol 2001; 124(1):62–68.

Reybrouck T, Fagard R. Gender differences in the oxygen transport system during maximal exercise in hypertensive subjects. Chest 1999; 115:788–792.

Richman RA, Sheehe PR, McCanty T, Vespasiano M, Post EM, Guzi S, Wright H. Olfactory deficits in boys with cleft palate. Pediatrics 1988; 82(6):840–844.

Rifkind BM, Schucker B, Gordon DJ. When should patients with heterozygous familial hypercholesterolemia be treated? JAMA 1999; 281(2):180–181.

Robinson GE. Women and psychopharmacology. Medscape Women's Health eJournal 2002; 7(1).

Rodin J. Cultural and psychosocial determinants of weight concerns. Ann Intern Med 1993; 119(7 pt 2):643–645.

Roger VL, Farkouh ME, Weston SA, Reeder GS, Jacobsen SJ, Zinsmeister AR, Yawn BP, Kopecky SL, Gabriel SE. Sex differences in evaluation and outcome of unstable angina. JAMA 2000; 283(5):646–652.

Romani A, Bergamaschi R, Versino M, Delnevo L, Callieco R, Cosi V. Spinal and cortical potentials evoked by tibial nerve stimulation in humans: Effects of sex, age and height. Boll Soc Ital Biol Sper 1992; 68(11):691–698.

Romanzi LJ. Urinary incontinence in women and men. J Gend Specif Med 2001; 4(3):14–20.

Rosen CJ, Kessenich CR. Risk factors for osteoporosis in men: Prevention and treatment implications. Clinical Geriatrics 1997; 5(4):87–96.

Rosen EM. Prevent injuries America! Women's Health Orthopedic Edition 2000; 3(2):40.

Rosen EM. The bone and joint decade. Women's Health Orthopedic Edition 1999; 2(5):2.

Rosenfeld JA. Pharmacokinetics. The Female Patient 1997; 22:37–43.

Rowland T, Goff D, Martel L, Ferrone L. Influences of cardiac functional capacity on gender differences in maximal oxygen uptake in children. Chest 2000; 117(3):629–635.

Rubel, LR, Rabin L, Seeff LB, Licht H, Cuccherini BA. Does primary biliary cirrhosis in men differ from primary biliary cirrhosis in women? Hepatology 1984; 4(4):671–677.

Ruff CB, Hayes WC. Sex differences in age-related remodeling of the femur and tibia. J Orthop Res 1988; 6(6):886–896.

Sahd JA. Sexual identity of the nervous system. Rev Invest Clin 1989; 41(1):67–75.

Sahn SA, Heffner JE. Spontaneous pneumothorax. N Engl J Med 2000; 342(12):868–74.

Sakane T, Takeno M, Suzuki N, Inaba G. Behcet's disease. N Engl J Med 1999; 341(17):1284–1291.

Salo JA, Soisalon-Soininen S, Bondestam S, Mattila PS. Familial occurences of abdominal aortic aneurysm. Ann Intern Med 1999; 130(8):637–642.

Saltonstall R, Healthy bodies, social bodies:Men's and women's concepts and practices of health in everyday life. Soc Sci Med 1993; 36(1):7–14.

Sandler RS, Jordan MC, Shelton BJ. Demographic and dietary determinants of constipation in the US population. Am J Public Health 1990; 80(2):185–189.

Sandstede J, Lipke C, Beer M, Hofmann S, Pabst T, Kenn W, Neubauer S, Hahn D. Age- and gender-specific differences in left and right ventricular cardiac function and mass determined by cine magnetic resonance imaging. Eur Radiol 2000; 10(3):438–442.

Santilli JD, Santilli SM Diagnosis and treatment of abdominal aortic aneurysms. American Family Physician 1997; 56(4):1081–1090.

Sasaki R, Kurokawa T, Kobayasi T, Tero-Kubota S. Influences of sex and age on serum ascorbic acid. Tohoku J Exp Med 1983; 140(1):97–104.

Sato H, Sando I, Takahashi H. Sexual dimorphism and development of the human cochlea. Computer 3-D measurement. Acta Otolaryngol 1991; 111(6):1037–1040.

Schappert SM. Office visits to orthopedic surgeons:United States, 1995–96. Advance data from Vital and Health Statistics; No. 302. National Center for Health Statistics, Hyattsville, Md 1998; Publication (PHS) 98-1250.

Schauder P, Zavelberg D, Langer K, Herbertz L. Sex-specific differences in plasma branched-chain keto acid levels in obesity. Am J Clin Nutr 1987; 46(1):58–60.

Schellinger D, Lin CS, Fertikh D, Lee JS, Lauerman WC, Henderson F, Davis B. Normal lumbar vertebrae: Anatomic, age, and sex variance in subjects at proton MR spectroscopy—initial experience. Radiology 2000; 215(3):910–916.

Schleupner CJ. Urinary tract infections: Separating the genders and the ages. Postgraduate Medicine 1997; 101(6):231–237.

Schneider F, Habel U, Kessler C, Salloum JB, Posse S. Gender differences in regional cerebral activity during sadness. Hum Brain Mapp 2000; 9(4):226–238.

Schwartz BS, Stewart WF, Simon D, Lipton RB. Epidemiology of tension-type headache. JAMA 1998; 279(5):381–383.

Schwartz JB. Congestive heart failure medications: Is there a rationale for sex-specific therapy? J Gend Specif Med 2000; http//:www.mmhc.com/jgsm/articles/JGSM0008/schwartz.html.

Schwartz JB. Gender and dietary influences on drug clearance. J Gend Specif Med 2000; 3(2):30–37.

Schwartz JB. Gender differences in response to drugs: Pain medications. J Gend Specif Med 1999; 2(5):28–30.

Schwartz JB. The electrocardiographic QT Interval and its prolongation in response to medications: Differences between men and women. J Gend Specif Med 2000; 3(5):25–28.

Sebert P, Barthelemy L, Mialon P. CO_2 chemoreflex drive of ventilation in man: Effects of hyperoxia and sex differences. Respiration 1990; 57(4):264–267.

Seppa N. Secrets underlie lethal heart condition. Science News 1997; 152:155.

Sevre K, Lefrandt JD, Nordby G, Os I, Mulder M, Gans RO, Rostrup M, Smit AJ. Autonomic function in hypertensive and normotensive subjects: The importance of gender. Hypertension 2001; 37(6):1351–1356.

Shamim W, Yousufuddin M, Bakhai A, Coats AJ, Honour JW. Gender differences in the urinary excretion rates of cortisol and androgen metabolites. Ann Clin Biochem 2000; 37(Pt 6):770–774.

Shannon JR, Flattem NL, Jordan J, Jacob G, Black BK, Biaggioni I, Blakely RD, Robertson D. Orthostatic intolerance and tachycardia associated with norepinephrine-transporter deficiency. N Engl J Med 2000; 342(8):541–549.

Share L, Crofton JT, Ouchi Y. Vasopressin: Sexual dimorphism in secretion, cardiovascular actions and hypertension. Am J Med Sci 1988; 295(4):314–319.

Shelton DL. Survey looks at teaching trends in gender-based health issues. American Medical News May 5 1997:16.

Shephard RJ. Exercise and training in women, Part I: Influence of gender on exercise and training responses. Can J Appl Physiol 2000; 25(1):19–34.

Shulman KA, Berlin JA, Harless W, Kerner JF, Sistrunk S, Gersh BJ, Dube R, Taleghani CK, Burke JE, Williams S, Eisenberg JM, Escarce JJ. The effect of race and sex on physicians' recommendations for cardiac catheterization. N Engl J Med 1999; 340(8):618–626.

Simoneau JA, Bouchard C. Human variation in skeletal muscle fiber-type proportion and enzyme activities. Am J Physiol 1989; 257(4 Pt 1):E567–E572.

Simoni-Wastila L. The use of abusable prescription drugs: The role of gender. J Womens Health Gend Based Med 2000; 9(3):289–297.

Sinaki M, Nwaogwugwu NC, Phillips BE, Mokri MP. Effect of gender, age and anthropometry on axial and appendicular muscle strength. Am J Phys Med Rehabil 2001; 80(5):330–338.

Singh JP, et al. Reduced heart rate variability and new-onset hypertension: Insights into pathogenesis of hypertension: The Framingham Heart Study; Hypertension 1998; 32:293–297.

Singh R, Weigers SE, Goldstein BJ. Impact of gender on diabetes mellitus and its associated cardiovascular risk factors. J Gend Specif Med 2001; 4(3):28–36.

Siriwat PP, Jarabak JR. Malocclusion and facial morphology is there a relationship? An epidemiologic study. Angle Orthod 1985; 55(2):127–138.

Small GW. Estrogen effects on the brain. J Gend Specif Med 1998; 1(2):23–27.

Smit E, et al. Estimates of animal and plant protein intake in US Adults: Results from the Third National Health and Nutrition Examination Survey, 1988–1991. Journal of the American Dietetic Association 1999; 99:813–820.

Smulyan H, Asmar RG, Rudnicki A, London GM, Safar ME. Comparative effects of aging in men and women on the properties of the arterial tree. J Am Coll Cardiol 2001; 37(5):1374–1380.

Snow KK, Seddon JM. Age-related eye diseases: Impact of hormone replacement therapy, and reproductive and other risk factors. Int J Fertil 2000; 45(5):301–313.
Sonzogni JJ Jr. Sports injuries in female athletes, Part I. Emergency Medicine 2000; 32(5)60–76.
Sonzogni, JJ Jr. Sports injuries in female athletes, Part II: Common acute shoulder disorders. Emergency Medicine 2000; 32(6)62–81.
Soravia-Dunand VA, Loo VG, Salit IE. Aortitis due to salmonella: Report of 10 cases and comprehensive review of the literature. Clinical Infectious Diseases 1999; 29:862–868.
Sorensen M, Rasmussen OO, Tetzschner T, Christiansen J. Physiological variation in rectal compliance. Br J Surg 1992; 79(10):1106–1108.
Span JP, Pieters GF, Sweep FG, Hermus AR, Smals AG. Gender differences in rhGH-induced changes in body composition in GH-deficient adults. J Clin Endocrinol Metab 2001; 86(9):4161–4165.
Spierer A, Isenberg SJ, Inkelis SH. Characteristics of the iris in 100 neonates. J Pediatr Ophthalmol Strabismus 1989; 26(1):28–30.
Staron RS, Hagerman FC, Hikida RS, Murray TF, Hostler DP, Crill MT, Ragg KE, Toma K. Fiber type composition of the vastus lateralis muscle of young men and women. J Histochem Cytochem 2000; 48(5):623–629.
Sterling TRVlahov D, Astemborski J, Hoover DR, Margolick JB, Quinn TC. Initial plasma HIV-1 RNA levels and progression to AIDS in women and men; N Engl J Med 2001; 344:720–725.
Stevens GH, Graham TE, Wilson BA. Gender differences in cardiovascular and metabolic responses to cold and exercises. Can J Physiol Pharmacol 1987; 65(2):165–171.
Stewart JH, McCormick WF. The gender predictive value of sternal length. Am J Forensic Med Pathol 1983; 4(3):217–220.
Storstein L, Bjornstad H, Hals O, Meen HD. Electrocardiographic findings according to sex in athletes and controls. Cardiology 1991; 79(3):227–236.
Stroud CC, Marks RM. Management options for rheumatoid arthritis of the foot and ankle. Womens Health Orthopedic Edition; 1999; 2(5):30–35.
Sun LS. Gender differences in pain sensitivity and responses to analgesia. J Gend Specif Med 1998; 1(1):28–30.
Svenningsen S, Terjesen T, Auflem M, Berg V. Hip motion related to age and sex. Acta Orthop Scand 1989; 60(1):97–100.
Takekuma K, Ando F, Niino N, Shimokata H. Age and gender differences in skin sensory threshold assessed by current perception in community-dwelling Japanese. J Epidemiol 2000; 10(1 Suppl):S33–S38.
Takiyyuddin MA, Neunabb HP, Cervenja JH, Kennedy B, Dinh TQ, Ziegler MG, Baron AD, O'Connor DT. Ultradian variations of chromogranin A in humans. Am J Physiol 1991; 261(4 Pt 2):R939–R944.
Tanguay R, Demirjian A, Thibault HW. Sexual dimorphism in the emergency of the deciduous teeth. J Dent Res 1984; 63(1):65–68.

Targum SD, Marshall LE, Magac-Harris K, Martin D. TRH tests in a healthy elderly population. Demonstration of gender differences. J Am Geriatr Soc 1989; 37(6):533–536.

Tarnopolsky MA. Gender differences in metabolism; nutrition and supplements. J Sci Med Sport 2000; 3(3):287–298.

Taylor JR, Twomey LT. Sexual dimorphism in human vertebral body shape. J Anat 1984; 138 (Pt 2):281–286.

Ter RB. Gender differences in gastroesophageal reflux disease. J Gend Specif Med 2000; 3(2):42–44.

Thayer JF, Johnsen BH. Sex differences in judgement of facial affect: A multivariate analysis of recognition errors. Scand J Psychol 2000; 41(3):243–246.

Tur E. Physiology of the skin—Differences between women and men. Clinics in Dermatology 1997; 15:5–16.

Turkeltaub PC, Gergen PJ. Prevalence of upper and lower respiratory conditions in the US population by social and environmental factors: data from the second National Health and Nutrition Examination Survey, 1976–1980 (NHANES II). Annals of Allergy 1991; 67; 147–154.

Udry JR. Why are males injured more than females? Injury Prevention 1998; 4:94–95.

Ungemack JA. Patterns of personal health practice: Men and women in the United States. Am J Prev Med 1994; 10(1):38–44.

Urano T, Sumiyoshi K, Nakamura M, Mori T, Takada Y, Takada A. Fluctuation of tPA and PAI-1 antigen levels in plasma: Difference of their fluctuation patterns between male and female. Thromb Res 1990; 60(2):133–139.

Vaccarino V, Krumholz HM, Yarzebski J, Gore JM, Goldberg RJ. Sex differences in 2-year mortality after hospital discharge for myocardial infarction. Ann Intern Med 2001; 134(3):173–181.

Vaccarion V, Parson L, Every NR, Barron HV, Krumholz HM. Sex-based differences in early mortality after myocardial infarction. N Engl J Med 1999; 341(4):217–225.

Valdemarsson S, Edvinsson L, Hedner P, Ekman R. Hormonal influence on calcitonin gene-related peptide in man: Effects of sex difference and contraceptive pills. Scand J Clin Lab Invest 1990; 50(4):385–388.

Veldhuis JD, Neuroendocrine control of pulsatile growth hormone release in the human: Relationship with gender. Growth Horm IGF Res 1998; 8(Suppl B):49–59.

Verdecchia P, Schillaci G, Boldrini F, Guerrieri M, Porcellati C. Sex, cardiac hypertrophy and diurnal blood pressure variations in essential hypertension. J Hypertens 1992; 10(7):683–692.

Villablanca AC. Coronary heart disease in women-Gender differences and effects of menopause. Postgraduate Medicine 1996; 100(3):191–194.

Vine MF, Stein L, Weigle K. Gender differences in responses to the Multitest CMI skin test in the general population. Ann Allergy Asthma Immunol 2000; 84:445–450.

Vittecoq O, Said LA, Michot C. Evolution of chronic recurrent multifocal osteitis toward spondyloarthropathy over the long term. Arthritis Rheum 2000; 43:109–119.

Wagtmans MJ, Verspaget HW, Lamers CB, van Hogezand RA. Gender-related differences in the clinical course of Crohn's disease. Am J Gastroenterol 2001; 96(5):1541–1546.

Ward MM, Studenski S. Systemic lupus erythematosus in men: A multivariate analysis of gender differences in clinical manifestations. J Rheumatol 1990; 17(2):220–224.

Washington DL, Bird CE. Sex differences in disease presentation in the emergency department. Ann Emerg Med 2002; 40:461–463.

Wauters M, Van Gaal L. Gender differences in leptin levels and physiology: A role for leptin in human reproduction. J Gend Specif Med 1999; 2(5):46–51.

Weil MD, Lamborn K, Edwards MSB, Wara WM. Influence of a child's sex on medulloblastoma outcome. JAMA 1998; 279:1474–1476.

Weinstock MA. The epidemic of squamous cell carcinoma. JAMA 1989; 262(15):2138–2140.

Wenger N, Speroff L, Packard B. Cardiovascular health and disease in women. N Eng J Med 1993; 329(4):247–256.

Wever RA. Sex differences in human circadian rhythms: Intrinsic periods and sleep fractions. Experientia 1984; 40(11):1226–1234.

Wexler LF. Studies of acute coronary syndromes in women-lessons for everyone. N Engl J Med 1999; 341(4):275–276.

Whitacre CC, Reingold SC, O'Looney PA, and the Task Force on Gender, Multiple Sclerosis and Autoimmunity. A gender gap in autoimmunity. Science 1999; 283:1277–1278.

White DP, Douglas NJ, Piclett CK, Weil JV, Zwillich CW. Sexual influences on the control of breathing. J Appl Physiol 1983; 54(4):874–879.

Wingard DL, The sex differential in morbidity, mortality, and lifestyle. Annu Rev Public Health 1984; 5:433–458.

Wilkerson RD, Mason MA. Differences in men's and women's mean ankle ligamentous laxity. Iowa Orthop J 2000; 20:46–48.

Williams AB, Cheetham MJ, Bartram CI, Halligan S, Kamm MA, Nicholls RJ, Kmiot WA. Gender differences in the longitudinal pressure profile of the anal canal related to anatomical structure as demonstrated on three-dimensional anal endosonography. Br J Surg 2000; 87(12):1674–1679.

Williams GH, Fisher ND, Hunt SC, Jeunemaitre X, Hopkins PN, Hollenberg NK. Effects of gender and genotype on the phenotypic expression of nonmodulating essential hypertension. Kidney Int 2000; 57(4):1404–1407.

Williams MR, Choudhri AF, Morales DLS, Helman DN, Oz MC. Gender differences in patients undergoing coronary artery bypass surgery, from a mandatory statewide database. J Gend Specif Med 2000; 3(1):41–48.

Williamson DF. Descriptive epidemiology of body weight and weight changes in U.S. adults. Ann of Intern Med 1993; 119:646–649.

Wilson JA, Pryde A, Macintyre CC, Maran AG, Heading RC. The effects of age, sex, and smoking on normal pharyngoesophageal motility. Am J Gastroenterol 1990; 85(6):686–691.

Wimmer M, Luttringer C, Colombi M. Enzyme activity patterns of phospoenolpyruvate carboxykinase, pyruvate kinase, glucose-6-phosphate-dehydrogenase and malic enzyme in human liver. Histochemistry 1990; 93(4):409–415.

Winer N, Sowers JR, Weber MA. Gender differences in vascular compliance in young, healthy subjects assessed by pulse contour analysis. J Clin Hypertense (Greenwich) 2001; 3(3):145–152.

Wisniewski AB, Sexually-dimorphic patterns of cortical asymmetry, and the role for sex steroid hormones in determining cortical patterns of lateralization. Psychoneuroendocrinology 1998; 23(5):519–547.

Witelson SF, Kigar DL. Sylvian fissure morphology and asymmetry in men and women: Bilateral differences in relation to handedness in men. J Comp Neurol 1992; 323(3):326–340.

Woda A, Pionchon P. A unified concept of idiopathic orofacial pain: Pathophysiologic features. J Orofac Pain 2000; 14(3):196–212.

Wolbrette D, Patel H. Arrhythmias and women. Curr Opin Cardiol 1999; 14(1):36–43.

Wolfe F, Cathey MA, Roberts FK. The latex test revisited. Rheumatoid factor testing in 8,287 rheumatic disease patients. Arthritis Rheum 1991; 34(8):951–960.

Wong TY, Klein R, Sharrett AR, Duncan BB, Couper DJ, Tielsch JM, Klein BEK, Hubbard LD. Retinal arteriolar narrowing and risk of coronary heart disease in men and women. The atherosclerosis risk in communities study. JAMA 2002; 287(9):1153–1159.

Wyller TB. Stroke and gender; J Gend Specif Med 1999; 2(3):41–45.

Xander HT, Wehrens MD, vos MA, Doevendans PA, Wellens HJ. Novel insights in the congenital long QT syndrome. N Eng J Med 2002; 137 (12):981–992.

Yamamoto A, Serizawa S, Ito M, Sato Y. Fatty acid composition of sebum wax eaters and urinary androgen level in normal human individuals. J Dermatol Sci 1990; 1(4):269–276.

Yanovski JA, Yanovski SZ, Sovik KN, Nguyen TT, O'Neil PM, Sebring NG. A prospective study of holiday weight gain. N Engl J Med 2000; 342(12):861–867.

Youdas JW, Garrett TR, Suman VJ, Bogard CL, Hallman HO, Carey JR. Normal range of motion of the cervical spine: An initial goniometric study. Phys Ther 1992; 72(11):770–780.

Young EA. Sex differences and the HPA axis: Implications for psychiatric disease. J Gend Specif Med 1998; 1(1):21–27.

Yucel M, Stuart GW, Maruff P, Velakoulis D, Crowe SF, Savage G, Pantelis C. Hemispheric and gender-related differences in the gross morphology of the anterior cingulate/paracingulate cortex in normal volunteers: An MRI morphometric study. Cereb Cortex 2001; 11(1):17–25.

Yue NC, Arnold AM, Longstreth WT Jr, et al. Sulcal, ventricular and white matter changes at MR imaging in the aging brain: Data from the Cardiovascular Health Study. Radiology 1997; 202:33–39.

Yunus MB. Gender differences in fibromyalgia and other related syndromes. J Gen Specif Med 2002; 5(2):42–47.

Zeiner AR, Kegg PS, Blackburn M, Stratton R. Gender differences in peak acetaldehyde concentration after an acute dose of ethanol. Neurobehav Toxicol Teratol 1983; 5(2):201–204.

Zeng SM, Yankowitz J, Widness JA, Strauss RG. Etiology of differences in hematocrit between males and females: Sequence-based polymorphisms in erythropoietin and its receptor. J Gend Specif Med 2001; 4(1):35–40.

Zhou M, Goto N, Goto J, Moriyama H, He HJ. Gender dimorphism of axons in the human lateral corticospinal tract. Okajimas Folia Anat Jpn 2000; 77(1):21–27.

Zietz B, Hrach S, Scholmerich J, Straub RH. Differential age-related changes of hypothalamus-pituitary-adrenal axis hormones in healthy women and men-role of interleukin 6. Exp Clin Endocrinol Diabetes 2001; 109(2):93–101.